THE
CANNABIS SPA
AT HOME

THE
CANNABIS SPA
AT HOME

How to Make Marijuana-Infused Lotions,
Massage Oils, Ointments,
Bath Salts, Spa Nosh, and More

SANDRA HINCHLIFFE

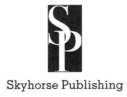

Skyhorse Publishing

Skyhorse Publishing books may be purchased in bulk at special discounts for sales promotion, corporate gifts, fund-raising, or educational purposes. Special editions can also be created to specifications. For details, contact the Special Sales Department, Skyhorse Publishing, 307 West 36th Street, 11th Floor, New York, NY 10018 or info@skyhorsepublishing.com.

Skyhorse® and Skyhorse Publishing® are registered trademarks of Skyhorse Publishing, Inc.®, a Delaware corporation.

Visit our website at www.skyhorsepublishing.com.

10 9 8 7 6 5 4 3 2

Library of Congress Cataloging-in-Publication Data is available on file.

Cover design by Laura Klynstra
Cover photos by Sandra Hinchliffe

Print ISBN: 978-1-5107-4088-4
Ebook ISBN: 978-1-5107-0057-4

Printed in the United States of America

For spa lovers everywhere.

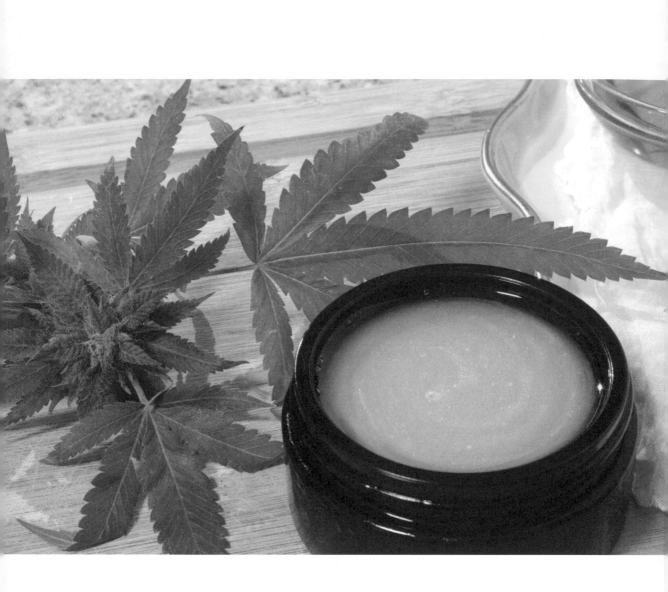

TABLE OF CONTENTS

Chapter Two: Lotions, Creams, and Scrubs   51

Cannabis lotion, creams, and scrubs are some of the best ways to enjoy the healing and beauty benefits of externally applied cannabis, without experiencing psychoactive side effects.

Chapter Three: Let's Get High on Bath Salts   75

There. I knew that would get your attention! But, I'm not talking about THOSE bath salts. Cannabis won't turn you into a zombie. I promise!

Chapter Four: Let's Get Well on Wraps, Masks, and Poultices   103

Cannabis works with wraps, masks, and poultices in ways that are similar to lotions and balms. The difference lies in their ability to be more spot-intensive, and you get the added benefits of detoxifying clay and additional healing herbs in these recipes.

Chapter Five: Aromatherapy, Tea, Bhang, and Smoothies   113

Delicious things for your spa day or any day! Try these along with other treatments, like a bath or massage, for a truly luxurious cannabis spa experience.

ACKNOWLEDGMENTS

Thanks to my husband, Greg, for his l33t hacking, bugfixing, proofreading, and housecleaning. Thanks to my agent, Rita Rosenkranz of Rita Rosenkranz Literary Agency, for seeing this project through, and all of the personal guidance she's given to a first-time author. Thanks to my fabulous editor and champion of this book, Nicole Frail at Skyhorse Publishing.

Personal Thanks:
My friend Rebecca at Therapy in a Bottle for her kind support; my friend Janet for her feedback on many of these recipes; my friend and sometimes coauthor at Hempista.com, Alisia, for her support and feedback. And thanks to all of the fans of this book and cannabis spa for your feedback and support!

PREFACE

This book is about the cannabis plant.

This book will demonstrate how to use cannabis to make you look and feel great, drawing from new and old traditions. It's a book about healing and elegance.

Because cannabis may be illegal in your location at the time of publication, some of the techniques and recipes in this book are only recommended for those in areas where cannabis is legal for general or medicinal purposes.

Please consult your local regulations or attorney for advice before trying the recipes and techniques described herein.

Also consult your personal doctor for health information and diagnosis. This book is not intended to diagnose or treat any illness and is not intended for pregnant or nursing mothers.

Nothing in this book is approved by the FDA or any other government agency.

This book is intended for mature readers, twenty-one years of age and older.

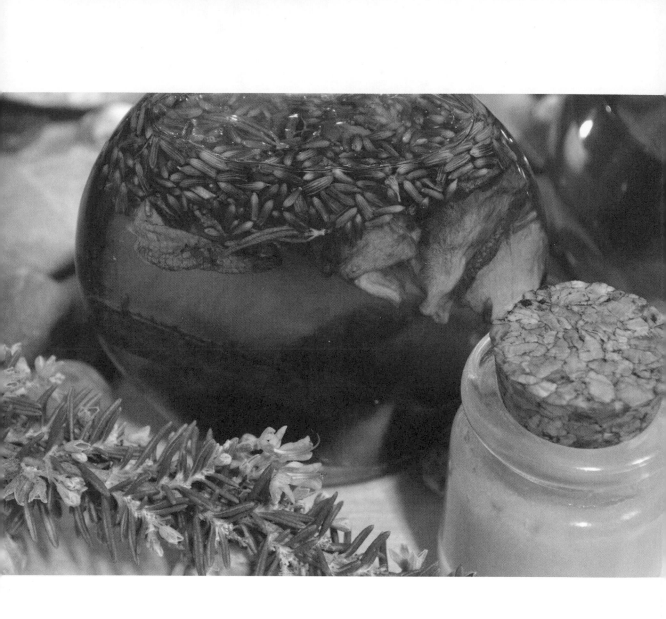

A NOTE FROM THE AUTHOR

Since 2011, I have been writing about cannabis spa and making my own cannabis spa formulations for refreshment, relaxation, and pain management. In 2013, I self-published a book about cannabis spa based on the very popular homemade cannabis lotions and spa potions featured on my website, hempista.com. Over the past two years, I've received a lot of great feedback and completed additional work developing wholesome new formulations—ranging from simple to lush and complex—for this expanded edition of *The Cannabis Spa at Home*.

I am thankful for the doctors and the medical science that saved my life when I was diagnosed with several autoimmune diseases; however, as an autoimmune patient, I feel there is one gigantic aspect of my illness that medical science failed to cure or even manage in a significant way—chronic pain. Furthermore, the staggering amount of pharmaceutical drug dependence in the United States tells me that medical science has also failed to adequately manage chronic pain for many others. I know I am not alone.

This is why I am passionate about the practice of spa—a centuries-old health practice across many cultures—as a path to sustainable relief from chronic pain. Cannabis is a nontoxic and easily cultivated herb that will add new dimensions to your spa experience, including skin healing properties, mind/body/soul refreshment, soothing analgesia, and anti-inflammatory effects.

I was first introduced to topical-use cannabis products through a legal cannabis medical collective, and I've been a huge fan ever since. One very attractive benefit of external cannabis products is their ability to provide cannabis medication without the "high" that you receive from vaporizing or ingesting cannabis orally. This was a lifesaver for work and drive time when getting high is not an option and is immediately beneficial as an effective adjunct to vaped or ingested cannabis when I needed more intensive pain management.

I use topical cannabis preparations daily, so I need a fresh product that is free of preservatives and allergens. As an anaphylactic allergy patient, I must carry an epinephrine pen in case of life-threatening allergic reactions, and quite often the commercially available external cannabis products did not meet my needs.

So I began making my own lotions, balms, baths, and everything in-between. In the process, I discovered that the cannabis herb has so many useful applications for wellness—beyond the vaporizer or the brownie! My experiments with herbal spa formulations using the cannabis plant became the recipes that I would regularly rely on, share with others, and write about.

For those who are beginners, my recipes stick mostly to basic food-grade ingredients that are easy to find and work with. And for the advanced external preparations folks who would like to try out new techniques and materials for their existing repertoire, I've included some techniques that are totally unique to this book and never before written about.

If you suffer from allergies or sensitivities, this book is for you! All the recipes in this book are free of major allergens such as eggs, soy, tree nuts, peanuts, fish, sesame, shellfish, yeast, mold, wheat, corn, latex, gluten, and dairy. (Please consult your doctor for allergy diagnosis and information on any of the ingredients if you are in doubt.)

Because this is a spa book, I've also included some of my favorite recipes for hemp smoothies and cannabis-medicated beverages called "bhang." I also enjoy cannabis aromatherapy, so I've included recipes for beautiful essence waters and cannabis aromatherapy techniques.

There are many ways to enjoy the beautiful cannabis herb, and it is my hope that you find my recipes so useful that you'll incorporate them into your wellness lifestyle.

AN INTRODUCTION TO CANNABIS

Cannabis is a genus of flowering plants in the family of *Cannabaceae*, which includes hops and the hackberry tree. Within the cannabis genus are three primary variations, *cannabis sativa*, *cannabis indica*, and *cannabis ruderalis*. Cannabis is native to regions of Asia and the first use of the plant for medicinal and general purposes is recorded there.

Cannabinoids

Cannabinoids are the active medicinal chemicals in the cannabis plant. Only one of these chemicals is known to cause the primary psychoactive effects, THC. There are sixty-plus cannabinoids in cannabis, including THC, THCA, THCV, CBG, CBN, CBC, and CBD.

In addition to THC—the cannabinoid responsible for that "high" feeling when you vape or ingest cannabis—the plant may also contain a significant amount of CBD, a non-psychoactive cannabinoid that has many healing applications including pain relief, inflammation relief, and anxiety relief. CBD has also been shown to be effective in controlling seizures in many patients.

Please consult your legal dispensary or grower for strains that have been tested for cannabinoid levels and then select the best strain for your needs based on this information.

Strains

This is a very informal guide to understanding the variations of the cannabis plant you will encounter. The cannabis spa recipes in this book are effective with any strain of cannabis rich in cannabinoids.

Cannabis sativa is a tall and skinny plant with elongated leaves. This variety may be medicinally active or it may be the variety that is also known as *hemp*. Hemp is non-psychoactive and bred in particular for its fiber (which can be made into many products) and its production of a seed that is highly nutritious in its raw state. Hemp also makes a lush, green, edible oil that is legal in every state and sold at natural food stores. Hemp is a variety of cannabis sativa that is industrial-grade and low in THC, making it legal to grow now in many places around the world, including Canada, China, Europe, and some parts of the United States.

When cannabis sativa is grown for medicinal purposes, the effects are heady and energetic. It can also relieve pain if it has a good percentage of naturally occurring CBD along with THC. In my personal opinion, high-CBD sativas provide the greatest amount of pain relief compared to any other strain—unless I want to sleep!

Cannabis indica is a short and broad leaf plant that can also express a range of purple, blue, and pink colors. Cannabis indica is always noted for its powerful cannabinoid content (up to 20 percent THC) and has been used for thousands of years in Asia and the Middle East for making concentrated hashishes that can be 50 percent or more THC total weight. Don't believe it if someone tells you "pot is stronger nowadays"—it's simply not true! The powerful cannabis indica plant has been used for thousands of years in concentrated form, much longer than prohibition has existed.

Cannabis indica has sleep-inducing and narcotic properties, which make it a great choice for evening pain control or relaxation. Its naturally occurring CBD enhances the other qualities of the plant as well.

Cannabis ruderalis is a small plant without many of the qualities of the other two primary variations of cannabis. This variety is used mostly for breeding purposes and isn't referenced in the recipes in this book unless it's part of the genetics of a hybrid variety.

Hybrid cannabis is very prevalent—most cannabis is hybrid today. Although landrace strains remain a favorite with many connoisseurs, the hybrids have some interesting variations, flavors, and colors that make them very popular.

Usually the hybrid will have most of the effects of the dominant strain; if there is more sativa than indica, the hybrid might be a bit more heady and vice versa. A great hybrid is one that has a nice balance between the two. Not too sleepy, not too heady, and just the right amount of pain relief.

Cannabis Plant Products Used in Cannabis Spa

Whole cured cannabis flowers contain terpenes, in addition to cannabinoids, in greater concentration than any of the processed forms of the cannabis flower. The flowers will retain their fragrant qualities and impart them to your cannabis spa preparations if they are carefully stored before use.

Here's something useful to consider when you are selecting a cannabis flower for an external-use: match the fragrance of the flower as close as possible to the fragrance profile of your preparation. For example, a cookie-flavored cannabis strain would pair well with a vanilla and cinnamon salve or lotion, while lemon or floral cannabis strains would work the best with rose creams.

Hashish is traditionally made by shaking, extracting, or rolling the resinous trichomes from mature cannabis flowers grown for their medicinal qualities. This technique concentrates the cannabinoids into a crumbly powder or a resin ball.

Keif is made by gently shaking off trichomes from cannabis flowers grown for their medicinal purposes. It is fluffy and powdery. Although it is a concentrated form of cannabinoids, it tends to have less potency than hashish, but more potency than the whole dried flower.

Trim are the leaves trimmed from the buds and the plant. These leaves contain the potent cannabinoids in smaller amounts than the flowers, so they're great for recipes in which you don't really care about the heavy green coloration from the chlorophyll.

Whole, fresh cannabis flowers and plants are full of vitality and healing! If you have access to fresh, live cannabis plants, you can create salves, lotions, and baths infused with the unique cannabinoid profile of fresh, live plant material.

Full-extract cannabis oil, otherwise known as Simpson Oil, is a whole herb extract of cannabis made through an alcohol distillation process that evaporates away the alcohol. This is an already decarboxylated cannabis product, unlike hashish, keif, or cannabis flowers, so it does not require heating to activate.

Prepare Cannabis Spa with Your Favorite Strains

All of these forms of cannabis are used in the recipes in this book, and each recipe can be prepared with whatever form of cannabis you have available. The recipes are not strain-specific, so it's a good idea to select the strains that you find the most beneficial. I've always prepared my spa potions and lotions with the highest quality clean cannabis herb available, which is also high in THC with a nice balance of CBD and other cannabinoids. I'm not crazy about spa preparations made with just one cannabinoid, such as "CBD only," which has exploded into a questionable market outside of the states that have legalized the whole herb for general and medicinal purposes.

Decarboxylation is the process of heating or aging cannabinoids so that they drop a carbon atom from their molecule. For example, decarboxylation of THCA is responsible for creating the psychoactive THC. Cannabinoids are useful in both their raw and decarboxylated state, but for most of the spa recipes in this book I use cannabis that has been heated or aged (decarboxylated).

Dr. Sanjay Gupta is correct, in my experience, when he said that the cannabis herb needs the "entourage effect" (the influence of a variety of cannabinoids, terpenes, and other plant constituents) to be the most effective. Help yourself and simply enjoy the luxury of cannabis spa by exploring these recipes using whole plant herbal medicine.

Authentic Cannabis Spa

Salves, lotions, and other spa preparations rich in cannabinoids, terpenes, and other plant constituents are the foundation of the spa philosophy behind this book. Cannabis is a virtually nontoxic herb with upward limits that would be difficult to reach—it's safe and satisfying to really get creative with cannabis spa potions and other external preparations!

Will I feel euphoric or "high" after applying cannabis topically?
Will I test positive on a drug test?

Typically, spa preparations will have no psychoactive effect when applied to your skin. But for your own peace of mind, you should always assume that if you are using cannabis in any form, you will test positive on a drug test.

Your local pharmacy will usually stock home-use drug tests; these are considered accurate enough to sell over the counter, but you should always consult a doctor and professional lab for more accurate drug testing.

There are instances where ointments and other topical preparations could become mildly psychoactive, such as in combination with soaking baths or by coming into contact with mucous membranes. Many of the spa preparations in this book are made with food-grade ingredients so they are also edible! Ingesting topical oils orally is similar to ingesting cannabis butter, or any other prepared culinary cannabis oil, in terms of its psychoactive effects and positive results on drug screening tests.

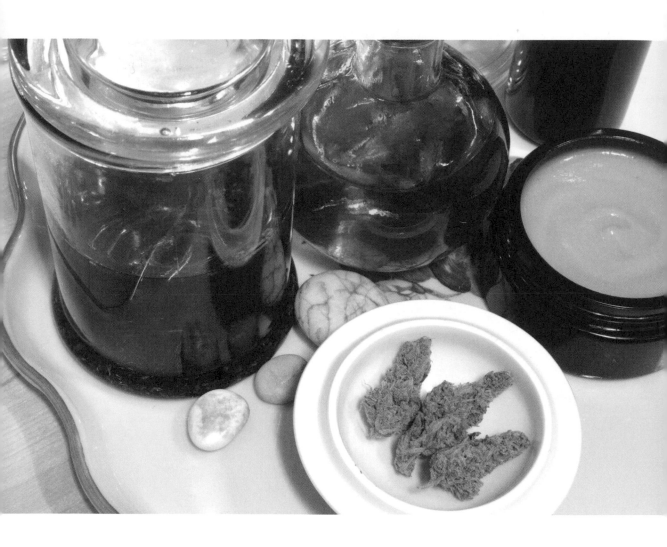

THE QUICK START GUIDE

Get relief, right now, right from your cupboard!

In the process of putting together this guide, it occurred to me that successful pain relief and relaxation with cannabis spa begins by learning simple techniques using ingredients that you have in your cupboard right now. Once you get comfortable with these techniques, the more complex recipes presented later in the book will help you explore new ways of working with and experiencing the cannabis herb.

Quick Start Ingredients

Olive oil is an ingredient most people have in their kitchen. It's also one of the most effective fats for use with external cannabis preparations. Olive oils higher in oleic acid work best to deliver deep penetration of the topical ingredients. Many nineteenth-century topical herbal medicines included oleic acids, and in my experiments, these fats absorb faster and more completely than other fatty acid profiles. Any kind of pure olive oil will work, but the type that contains the highest amount of oleic acid is typically a fresh, cold-pressed extra-virgin or virgin olive oil. High quality olive oils may have a cloudy appearance and a peppery or fruity taste.

I use a special technique with olive oil that I've found to be an exquisite method for creating a salve or ointment without adding any other fats or waxes: cold processing in the freezer or refrigerator. Olive oil is quite versatile. It can be made into a massage oil, ointment, or salve with the application of freezing or refrigeration. Cold-processing olive oil in the freezer produces a solid, cold salve, while in the refrigerator it produces a softer ointment. But this technique only works with pure olive oil, so for the best results, do not substitute olive oil or use an oil blend in the recipes in this chapter.

Cinnamon (powder or stick), ginger powder, turmeric powder, cloves, black pepper, and cayenne pepper powder are common spices found in many kitchens. They are noted for their warming and anti-inflammatory benefits, as well as for their lovely, natural fragrances.

Salt is used in the bath and plunge recipes. I use a high-quality, mineral-rich ancient sea salt or Himalayan salt, but you can use Epsom, Kosher, or even plain salt that has not been enriched with iodine.

Cut lemons, oranges, ginger root, turmeric root, fresh mint, parsley, thyme, and other common fresh and dried green herbs that you may have in your kitchen right now. These will have cooling or warming properties depending on how they are used in the recipes.

Clean towels and cloths using any absorbent fabric, hemp, or cotton is fine. You'll want a few sizes of towels and washcloths when doing the wraps.

Hot water, cold water, ice, and heat packs are used with the wraps and soaks.

Cannabis in trim, keif, or ground flower are the most effective forms for these recipes. You can make a highly effective and concentrated cannabis topical preparation using as little as ⅛ ounce or 3.5 grams of ground flowers, or ¼ ounce or 7 grams of cannabis trim.

The less potent the cannabis, the more cannabis material you'll need to make an effective recipe. These recipes are rich in cannabinoid content. For example: if you are using a highly potent flower, perhaps 18 percent or more THC and/or 10 percent or more CBD, approximately ⅛ ounce or 3.5–4 grams should be enough for each cup or 240 milliliters of olive oil. If you are using a lower potency flower, increasing the amount to 5–7 grams is ideal.

Alternatively, if you would like to use keif, 1–2 grams should be enough. Keif is one of my favorite forms of cannabis for use with these Quick Start salves and ointments because there is less chlorophyll and cannabis fragrance in the final product.

If you'd like to use more cannabis in your recipes than is suggested here, feel free to experiment! I've made successful batches of these recipes using up to an ounce of ground cannabis flowers. However, less is more when starting out, as you may find that the suggested amount—or even less—is the right amount for you.

Quick Start Salve, Ointment, and Massage Oil Recipes

These recipes are cold-processed either in the freezer for a solid salve preparation or in the refrigerator for a creamier ointment preparation. Both the salve and ointment melt easily into the skin. Cold-processing creates a cool and soothing sensation the minute the preparation is applied. Try it! You can also use any of these recipes in liquid form as massage oil, either chilled or warmed, prior to applying.

You may prepare these recipes two ways, and each way has advantages. The first, water processing of the oil in a pan on the stove or a slow cooker, will produce a fresher fragrance, eliminating some of the more pungent cannabis odors in the finished oil.

The alternate way to prepare the oil uses a canning jar filled with the oil and herbs, sealed, and then processed in a canning bath the way you would process jam or canned fruit. The oil will retain all of the cannabis fragrance. While the water processing method can be used with fresh or dried herbs, the canning jar processing method should only be used with dry herbs as it is important to keep moisture out of the final oil.

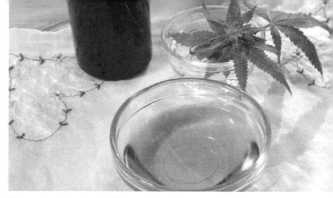

Warm olive oil and cannabis massage oil

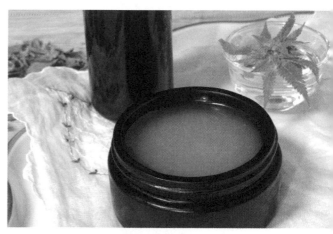

Soft and silky olive oil and cannabis refrigerator ointment

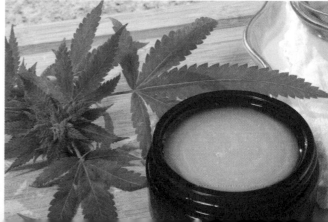

Firm and cool olive oil and cannabis freezer salve

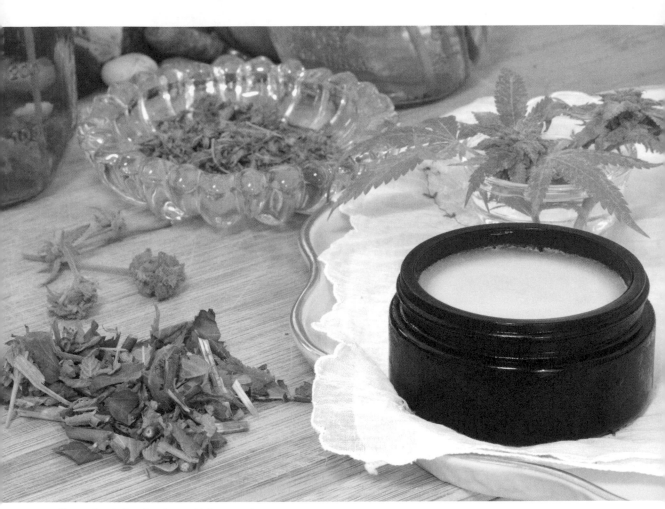

Firm and cool olive oil and cannabis freezer salve

Basic Quick Start Cannabis Salve, Ointment, or Massage Oil Recipe

1 cup (240 ml) olive oil
⅛ ounce (3.5 grams) or
more ground cannabis
flower
OR 1–2 grams or more
keif
OR ¼ ounce (7 grams)
cannabis trim or more,
chopped or ground
3 cups (720 ml) water for
the pan, rice cooker, or
slow cooker preparation
method—omit this
ingredient if you are
using the canning jar
processing method

This is the foundation recipe for all of the salve, ointment, and massage oil recipes in this chapter; all formulations in this chapter use the same oil extraction methods used in this Basic Quick Start recipe.

This recipe is specifically designed for sensitive skin, as it does not contain any of the supporting ingredients in the recipes that follow, such as cinnamon. This recipe has only two: olive oil and cannabis!

As a massage oil, this preparation is shelf-stable in a cool and dry area for up to six months. Store in freezer for salve or refrigerator for ointment.

Water and oil processing using a pan on the stove or slow cooker:

1. Pour the olive oil and cannabis material into the pan or cooker along with 3 cups or 720 milliliters of water and stir. If you are using additional herbs, as in the recipes that follow, add those to the pan or cooker along with the cannabis.
2. If you are using a pan on the stove, set on low heat and allow this to simmer slowly with the lid on for one hour. I've let this heat as long as two hours, but I think the final fragrance of the oil is better between the 60–90 minute mark.
3. If you are using a rice cooker, set for a normal brown rice cooking cycle, which should take 30–45 minutes. After the cooking cycle is complete, allow this to remain on warm for 30 minutes.
4. If you are using a slow cooker, set on low and cook for 4 hours.
5. It may be necessary to add additional water for longer cooking times, but typically 3 cups or 720 milliliters of water will last the entire cooking cycle. Do not allow the oil to burn or "fry" the plant matter, as this will change the fragrance and composition of the essential oils.
6. Line a strainer with three layers of cheesecloth and strain. Squeeze the last of the liquid from the plant material and set aside the plant material for additional recipes; the leftover plant material is great for hot and cool wraps and poultices.
7. After the oil and water have completely separated at room temperature, put the oil and water into the freezer for 1 hour or more and allow the oil to become very solid. Use a warm spoon or knife to separate the oil from the water, and spoon this oil into a clean container. Allow the oil to warm up to room temperature and then pour into a final container that has been sterilized in boiling water for fifteen minutes and dried.

Alternatively, you may siphon the oil from the top using a syringe after the oil and water have completely separated at room temperature. Siphon the oil and transfer it into the sterilized glass bottle or jar. It's important to ensure that water is not transferred to the sterile oil container. Leave a thin oil slick and siphon that up separately. Use this bit immediately as a moisturizing massage oil, as it will contain a small amount of herbal water from the oil-making process.

Canning jar preparation method:

1. In a canning jar, marinate the cannabis and other herbs—if you are using them—in olive oil until saturated. Leave at least 2 inches (5cm) at the top of the jar. Affix the lid tightly. Place in a canning bath or stock pan filled with water and simmer for 60–90 minutes on the stove. Check this frequently to ensure that the pan does not boil dry and add more water if necessary.

2. Remove from the stove and allow the jar to cool until it can be safely handled. Take care when unscrewing the lid as it may have become sealed during the processing of the oil. Strain the oil from the plant material through two or three layers of cheesecloth. Squeeze out as much of the oil as possible. Set aside the plant material to later use in the recipes that follow.

You may use the oil immediately, but the best way to enjoy this oil's benefits is by cold-storing it in the freezer to create a solid salve, in the refrigerator to create a creamy ointment, or on a shelf at room temperature for massage-oil consistency. If the oil has softened, you will want to stir the oil after each use before refrigerating again. This will always ensure a creamy and smooth application each time.

Olive oil absorbs easily into the skin after several minutes, so you can feel free to apply as much as you would like while massaging it in. Or you can leave a thicker layer on the skin for applications such as the hot and cold towel wraps and the soak and bath recipes.

Cinnamon Spiced Quick Start Cannabis Salve, Ointment, or Massage Oil

1 cup (240 ml) olive oil
3 cups (720 ml) water
for the pan, rice
cooker, or slow cooker
preparation method—
omit this ingredient
if you are using the
canning jar processing
method
⅛ ounce (3.5 grams) or
more ground cannabis
flower
OR 1–2 grams or more
keif
OR ¼ ounce (7 grams)
or more cannabis trim,
chopped or ground
2 teaspoons (4 grams)
powdered cinnamon
OR 5 cinnamon sticks

This recipe is just like the Basic Quick Start recipe, but with the addition of one of the most common and most medicinally effective spices in the kitchen: cinnamon. This oil is warming, and the cinnamon and cannabis penetrate deeply into sore tissues and joints.

Take care not to get this preparation into open wounds or in your eyes due to heat from the cinnamon. This recipe can be completed using either cinnamon sticks or powder. As a massage oil, this preparation is shelf-stable in a cool and dry place for up to six months. Store in freezer for salve or refrigerator for ointment.

Prepare this recipe using the **Basic Quick Start Cannabis Salve, Ointment, or Massage Oil Recipe** methods of oil preparation. This recipe is most effective when it is refrigerated and allowed to become a solid salve in the freezer or semi-soft ointment in the refrigerator before application.

Healing Spice Trinity Quick Start Cannabis Salve, Ointment, or Massage Oil

This recipe incorporates three common kitchen spices—cinnamon, ginger, and cayenne pepper—in a formula that is very warming and anti-inflammatory. Cayenne pepper, combined with cannabis in this recipe, provides potent pain relief. Similar to the Cinnamon Spiced Quick Start Cannabis Salve recipe, be sure to avoid getting this ointment in your eyes, other mucous membranes, or any open wounds because of the heat from these spices.

Prepare this recipe using the **Basic Quick Start Cannabis Salve, Ointment, or Massage Oil Recipe** methods of oil preparation. If you are using fresh ginger root in this recipe, use the pan, rice cooker, or slow cooker methods.

This oil is best frozen or refrigerated first so it will turn into a salve or ointment. Stir this oil after use and before refrigerating or freezing again for the best results.

1 cup (240 ml) olive oil

3 cups (720 ml) water for the pan, rice cooker, or slow cooker preparation method—omit this ingredient if you are using the canning jar processing method (use powdered or dried ginger only for this method)

⅛ ounce (3.5 grams) or more ground cannabis flower

OR 1–2 grams or more keif

OR ¼ ounce (7 grams) or more cannabis trim, chopped or ground

1 teaspoon (2 grams) powdered cinnamon

½ teaspoon (1 gram) cayenne pepper powder

1 tablespoon (5 grams) powdered ginger

OR ¼ cup (15 grams) grated fresh ginger

Shalimar Spice Quick Start Cannabis Salve, Ointment, or Massage Oil

1 cup (240 ml) olive oil

3 cups (720 ml) water for the pan, rice cooker, or slow cooker preparation method—omit this ingredient if you are using the canning jar processing method

⅛ ounce (3.5 grams) or more ground cannabis flower
OR 1–2 grams or more keif
OR ¼ ounce (7 grams) cannabis trim or more, chopped or ground

1 tablespoon (7 grams) dried clove buds

1 tablespoon (7 grams) black pepper

1 tablespoon (5 grams) turmeric
OR ¼ cup (15 grams) grated fresh turmeric root

Named after my favorite San Francisco Bay Area restaurant and the culinary spice traditions of Pakistan and India, this recipe includes three common kitchen spices: cloves, black pepper, and turmeric. I love this recipe for its ability to penetrate deeply into sore joints. But because it contains a lot of turmeric, this preparation will stain clothing and temporarily stain your skin a beautiful golden color (or glow if you have darker skin).

This recipe may be created using fresh turmeric roots if you have them handy, otherwise turmeric powder will work just fine.

Prepare this recipe using the **Basic Quick Start Cannabis Salve, Ointment, or Massage Oil Recipe** methods of oil preparation. If you are using fresh turmeric in this recipe, use the pan, rice cooker, or slow cooker methods.

Freeze or refrigerate to create a salve or ointment that can be easily applied. It is best to stir the oil if it softens before freezing or refrigerating again.

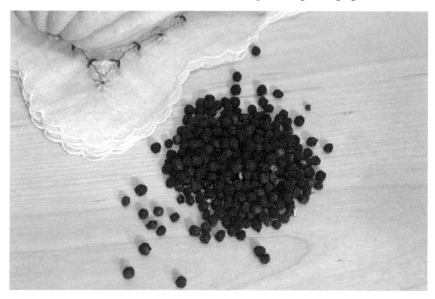

Cooling Herbs Healing Quick Start Cannabis Salve, Ointment, or Massage Oil

This recipe is for cooling relief of irritated skin and includes chamomile, mint, thyme, marjoram, and rosemary. I like to break open bags of chamomile tea and add it to dried mint, thyme, marjoram, and rosemary. This soothing and cooling skin salve was inspired by the "Four Thieves" formula of the Middle Ages using common European kitchen herbs. I like to use all five but if you only have two or three, plus the chamomile—which is essential to this recipe—you can still make a great salve, ointment, or massage oil with whatever herbs you have in your cupboard.

Prepare this recipe using the **Basic Quick Start Cannabis Salve, Ointment, or Massage Oil Recipe** methods of oil preparation.

The oil is ready to use if you need relief right away! However, like the other recipes, this oil is best frozen or refrigerated first so it solidifies into a salve or ointment. Stir this oil after use and before refrigerating again for the best results.

1 cup (240 ml) olive oil
3 cups (720 ml) water for the pan, rice cooker, or slow cooker preparation method—omit this ingredient if you are using the canning jar processing method (use this method with dried herbs only)
⅛ ounce (3.5 grams) or more ground cannabis flower
OR 1-2 grams or more keif
OR ¼ ounce (7 grams) or more cannabis trim, chopped or ground
2 tablespoons (3 grams) chamomile
2 tablespoons (3 grams) mint leaves
2 tablespoons (3 grams) thyme
2 tablespoons (3 grams) marjoram
2 tablespoons (3 grams) rosemary

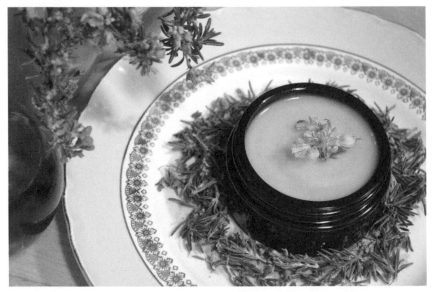

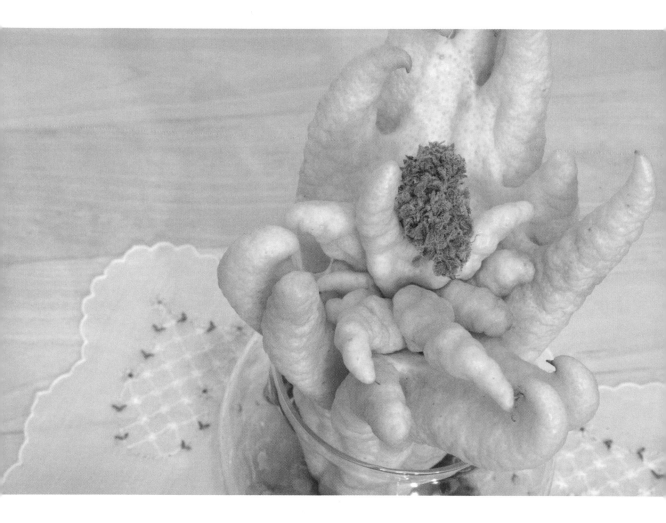

Fresh Fruits and Herbs Quick Start Cannabis Salve, Ointment, or Massage Oil

I've saved the best for last because with this Quick Start recipe you can get as creative as you want, infusing your favorite fresh fruit and herb blends to create a cannabis salve, ointment, or massage oil. If you are feeling a little more adventurous and want to indulge in a very euphoric experience, this recipe makes a delicious edible massage oil when prepared using your favorite fruit, flower, and herbal ingredients.

Here are some simple fruit and herb blends that I like to make with fresh ingredients:

Buddha's hand citron + roses + mint + cannabis

lime + rosemary + sage + cannabis

orange + basil + thyme + cannabis

You may also experiment using dried or fresh cannabis flowers and trim in this recipe. I have used each of these fresh ingredients, including fresh cannabis flowers, with fantastic results.

This recipe is also almost identical to the **Basic Quick Start Cannabis Salve, Ointment, or Massage Oil Recipe**, with a few modifications to infuse a generous amount of fresh ingredients all at once.

1. Pour the olive oil, chopped fresh ingredients, and cannabis material into the pan or cooker along with 1 quart (1 liter) of water, and stir.
2. If you are using a pan on the stove, set on low heat and allow this to simmer slowly with the lid on (do not boil) for 90 minutes.
3. If you are using a rice cooker, set for a normal brown rice cooking cycle, which should take 30–45 minutes. After the cooking cycle is complete, allow this to remain on warm for 60 minutes.
4. If you are using a slow cooker, set on low and cook for 4 hours.
5. Line a strainer with three layers of cheesecloth and strain. Squeeze the last of the liquid from the plant material and set aside the plant material for additional recipes; the leftover plant material is great for hot and cool wraps, scrubs, and poultices.

1 cup (240 ml) olive oil
4 cups (1 liter) water
⅛ ounce (3.5 grams) or
   more ground cannabis
   flower
   OR 1–2 grams or more
   keif
   OR ¼ ounce (7 grams)
   or more cannabis trim,
chopped or ground a
   generous assortment of
   your favorite chopped
   fruits, flowers, and
   herbs!*

6. After the oil and water have completely separated at room temperature, put the oil and water into the freezer for 1 hour or more and allow the oil to become very solid. Use a warm spoon or knife to separate the hard oil from the water, and spoon this oil into a clean container. Allow the oil to warm up to room temperature and then pour into a final container that has been sterilized in boiling water for 15 minutes and dried.

Alternatively, after the oil and water have completely separated at room temperature, you may siphon the oil from the top instead of freezing using a syringe. Siphon the oil and transfer it into the sterilized glass bottle or jar.

It's important to ensure that water is not transferred to the sterile oil jar, so leave a thin oil slick and siphon that up separately. Use it immediately as a moisturizing massage oil, as it will contain a small amount of herbal water from this oil-making process.

------

* Use as much as you like, as long as the water and oil completely cover all of the other ingredients with 1½ inches (4 cm) or more space at the top. If necessary, you can add more water during the cooking process.

Herbal Spa Oil Jar

If you are a fan of vaporizing cannabis flowers like I am, keeping an herbal spa oil jar is the perfect way to get the most out of your vaped cannabis flowers. Many people will use their leftover and toasted ground cannabis flowers in edible cannabis recipes because vaping cannabis never completely removes all of cannabinoids from the plant material. I use my vape tailings in a jar of selected medicinal herbs and oil, then age it a few months to create a medicinal cannabis topical oil, salve, or ointment.

Vape tailings have a "toasty" fragrance after being used in a vape and are brown in color. Don't use vape tailings that are black in color or those containing any ash whatsoever. Vape tailings a light to medium brown color are ideal for making this herbal oil preparation.

Vape tailings are already decarboxylated, so they are ready to use without any additional heating. All they need is time and the infused synergy from the other herbs to create an extraordinary massage oil, salve, or ointment using only olive oil.

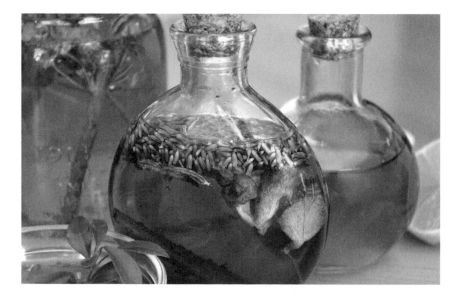

1 pint canning jar or other closed glass container like an apothecary jar
⅛ ounce (3.5 grams) or more toasted cannabis vape tailings
dried herbal assortment*
1–2 cups (240–480 ml) olive oil

Your first herbal oil vape jar can be as simple as the other recipes in this chapter, or it can be more complex—there's really no limit to the number of herbs and spices you can use. **Please consult labeling and reliable sources to determine the photosensitivity potential of each ingredient when selecting herbs and spices for your herbal oil jar.**

There are so many ways to get creative with your jar to create the herbal spa oil that is perfect for you. Remember, vape tailings have their own "toasty" fragrance that should play well with the other herbs you select. I have used the oil made with this herbal spa oil jar to make massage oil, ointment, and salves, but I wouldn't use this oil for the fresher spa preparations such as lotions, cold creams, or lotion bar recipes in the chapters that follow.

1.   Sterilize a glass jar with boiling water for 10 minutes. Allow this to dry and cool completely.
2.   Place your desired clean, dried herbs and spices in the jar along with cannabis vape tailings.
3.   Warm the olive oil to 200 degrees Fahrenheit (93 degrees Celcius), then pour this over the dried herbal mixture in the glass jar and shake. Place the jar away from heat and sunlight.

I like to age the contents of these jars for at least 1 month before straining out the oil and turning it into a salve in the freezer or into an ointment in the refrigerator. I've aged jars up to 6 months or longer using miron glass technology, which I will explain more about in the chapters that follow.

My herbal spa oil jar is rich and complex, and I continually add more vape tailings, oil, herbs and spices, and start new jars when the older jars reach their limits. I've poured this herbal spa oil into a clear glass jar from the miron glass apothecary jar, so you can see the herbal infusion. Lovely isn't it?

* Cinnamon sticks, cardamom pods, vanilla beans, dried marjoram, mint, thyme, turmeric, cayenne pepper, ginger, green tea, chamomile—it's your choice!

There are also resins like boswellia and additional dried herbs like rose petals, cinnamon, ginger, orange blossoms, mint, lavender, and more! Here are some common kitchen herb combinations you may enjoy trying with your new herbal spa oil jar:

vanilla pods + boswellia powder + cannabis = A sensual warm oil that is great for massage.

cinnamon sticks + ginger powder + turmeric powder + cannabis = A golden, tinted oil that is warming, anti-inflammatory, and pain relieving.

cayenne pepper + ginger powder + cloves + cannabis = A very warming oil for intensive pain relief. Great for muscle and nerve pain.

chamomile + mint + rosemary + cannabis = A cool skin-soothing oil for irritated skin. This herbal combination also makes a great massage oil or cold massage ointment.

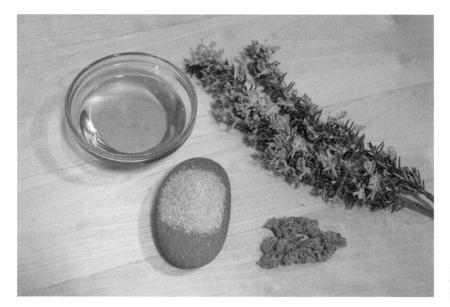

Clockwise from the bottom: cannabis, boswellia powder, olive oil, fresh rosemary flowers

Cannabis Herbal Scrub

leftover plant material from the **Quick Start** ointment recipes
½ cup (120 ml) olive oil
¼ cup (60 grams) salt or sugar, medium-coarse grind

One of the ways that you can use the leftover herbal mash when making any of the ointment recipes is to recycle the material into a scrub. This simple recipe should be kept refrigerated and used within one or two days. Try it before a bath for the best results.

1. Purée the plant material with the olive oil in a blender. Make sure as much liquid as possible has been squeezed from the plant material beforehand.
2. Pour the mixture into a clean glass jar, add the sugar or salt, and stir.
3. Put in the freezer immediately and allow this to remain for at least 1 hour. You may use the scrub immediately, but be sure to return it to the refrigerator after use. Keep refrigerated and use the scrub within two days for best results.

Quick Start Hot and Cold Soaks and Baths

Hot, Tired, Swollen Feet? Take the Cool Plunge!

This foot plunge is like putting your feet into an ice-cold mountain spring. It's very refreshing and perhaps a little shocking. Your hot, tired, and swollen feet will thank you!

There are more foot soak recipes in chapter 3 of this book, Getting High on Bath Salts, so you'll want to check those out, too, once you've mastered this quick start foot plunge technique.

1. Fill the spa or basin with cold water. Thoroughly dissolve the salt.
2. Massage a generous amount of the cannabis ointment into your feet and ankles.
3. Prepare your foot spa or basin with water and/or ice and lemon juice, then add the crushed mint leaves to the water.

After your feet have absorbed some of the oils from the cannabis ointment, about 15 minutes or so, you are ready to plunge them into the cold bath. Keep them there for as long as you like!

The Basic Quick Start Cannabis Salve, Ointment, or Massage Oil Recipe (page 5) a foot spa soaker or basin
¼ cup (60 grams) salt
cool to cold water*

* Optional but fabulous: juice from 1 fresh lemon and fresh mint that has been crushed a bit to release the essential oils directly into the water.

Painful Feet or Joints? Take the Warm Plunge!

Cinnamon Spiced, Healing Spice Trinity Quick Start Cannabis Salve, Ointment, or Massage Oil, or another warming spice ointment (page 7–8)

a foot spa soaker or basin
¼ cup (60 grams) salt
warm to hot-as-you-can-stand-it water* to fill the spa or basin.

This recipe works best when paired with any of the warming spice **Quick Start** ointments, salves, or massage oils.

1. Fill the spa or basin with water. Be sure to thoroughly dissolve the salt.
2. Massage a generous amount of the cannabis ointment into your feet and ankles.
3. Prepare your foot spa or basin with the heated water and the salt, then add the lemon juice and sliced ginger (if you so choose) to the water.

After your feet have absorbed some of the oils from the cannabis ointment, about 15 minutes, you are ready to plunge them into the warm foot bath.

Cool Off Now: The Full Body Fever Plunge

The Basic Quick Start Cannabis Salve, Ointment, or Massage Oil Recipe (page 5)
a tub filled with cool water
½ cup (125 grams) salt
2 cups (480 ml) hot water
1 large bunch of fresh mint
2 large sliced oranges

This is great for sunburn, fever, or any time you need to cool down right away.

1. Fill the bath with the salt and the coolest water temperature that is most comfortable for you.
2. In a blender, combine the hot water, mint leaves, and oranges. Blend until chopped, but not smooth, because you will want to strain this bath tea, especially if you are using a jet tub for your plunge. Strain the resulting bath tea and add to the bath water.
3. Generously apply the cannabis ointment to the heated areas of your body that need to cool down. Allow this to soak in for about 15 minutes before plunging into the bath.

* Optional but fabulous: juice from 1 fresh lemon and 1 large ginger root sliced and added directly to the hot water.

Warm Up Now: The Full Body Hot Plunge

This is my favorite **Quick Start** bath when I hurt literally everywhere. You'll want to adjust the temperature of this bath to be as hot as possible for the maximum benefit.

You can use any of the ointment recipes, but the best results are obtained with either the **Cinnamon Spiced**, **The Healing Spice Trinity Quick Start Cannabis Salve, Ointment, or Massage Oil**, or another warming spice ointment.

1. Generously apply the cannabis ointment to all areas that need relief. While this penetrates into your skin for 15 minutes, prepare the bath water with salt.
2. In a blender, coarsely blend the ginger, whole lemon, and hot water. Strain this bath tea and add to your bath. Plunge into your bath immediately!

The Quick Start Cannabis Salve, Ointment, or Massage Oil of your choice (page 5–10)
½ cup (125 grams) salt
1 large sliced ginger root *OR* 1 tablespoon (5 grams) ginger powder to substitute
1 lemon, cut in half
2 cups (480 ml) hot water

Painful Hands? Try the Quick Start Warm Hand Plunge!

Do you have arthritic or otherwise painful hands? Your hands will feel better within minutes using this warm hand plunge.

This recipe works best with any of the warming spice **Quick Start** ointments, salves, or massage oils and can be done in your sink.

1. Massage the ointment into your hands and allow 15 minutes to penetrate into the skin.
2. Prepare your sink or basin with warm to hot water and salt. Add the sliced ginger root and agitate. Plunge in your hands immediately!

The Quick Start Cannabis Salve, Ointment, or Massage Oil of your choice (page 5–10)
1 sink or basin full of warm to hot-as-you-can-stand-it water
¼ cup (60 grams) salt
1 large sliced ginger root *OR* 1 tablespoon (5 grams) ginger powder to substitute

Quick Start Wraps and Poultices

Wraps and poultices are a fast and intensive method of using cannabis topically. Many folk medicine practices include the use of wraps and poultices precisely because they are so quick and effective for applications such as pain relief. Traditional medicinal use of cannabis in Asia almost always includes the topical application of cannabis leaves.

Some of these recipes utilize the plant material leftovers from the quick start ointments. The leftover ingredients from the ointment recipes will be neatly packaged in the cheesecloth, after you have squeezed out all the liquid, and can be used as a poultice or wrap. Please note that that leftover trim or flower from the ointments that contain warming spices may irritate rashes and mucous membranes and shouldn't be used on any open wounds.

Quick Start Simple Cannabis Wrap—Hot or Cold, Your Choice!

The Basic Quick Start Cannabis Salve, Ointment, or Massage Oil Recipe (page 5)
3–4 clean towels
1 large pan or basin of ice water, including ice chips or cubes*

If you are experiencing heat and inflammation, chill down with this moist cooling wrap that uses the **Basic Quick Start Cannabis Salve, Ointment, or Massage Oil** Recipe.

1. Generously apply the cannabis ointment to the affected area.
2. Soak one towel in the ice water and squeeze. Wrap the cold towel around the affected area for 15–20 minutes.

If needed, cool the towel again in the ice water and reapply. For more intensive relief, ice packed inside of two cool, moist towels wrapped around the affected area is suggested. Adding brewed mint tea or crushing mint leaves in the ice water will add an additional cooling sensation to this wrap.

* Optional: add crushed mint leaves to the cold water

For the Hot Wrap

1. Apply the ointment generously to the affected area. If you are using hot water only, dip one towel in the water, squeeze, and apply immediately. Wrap an additional dry towel around the warm, wet towel. This should continue to produce heat for 15–20 minutes.

2. If you have heat packs or a heating pad, prepare a warm, moist towel the same way and wrap the affected area, placing the hot pack or heating pad on top of the warm, moist towel. Wrap this with a dry towel.

This wrap will provide heat for 30 minutes or more, or when you need a more intensive heat overall.

any of the **Quick Start** ointments*
3–4 clean towels
1 large pan or basin of hot water and/or hot packs or a moist heating pad

———

* For best results use any of the warming spice **Quick Start** ointments, salves, or massage oils.

Quick Start Warming Cannabis Poultice

My favorite way to use this poultice is on my arthritic hands, which are then covered with spa gloves that I've warmed in the dryer. It's also great for achy joints and muscles and can even be combined with head packs or wraps.

1. Put the cannabis material, ginger, and boiling water into the blender and blend until it is a smooth paste.

2. Apply this mixture to the desired area and wrap with clean gauze. Apply additional moist heat as needed.

leftover cannabis flower or trim material from any of the **Quick Start** ointments*
1 large sliced ginger root *OR* 2 tablespoons (10 grams) ginger powder to substitute
3 tablespoons (45 ml) boiling water
a blender
clean wrapping gauze

———

* The **Cinnamon Spiced** or the **Healing Spice Trinity Quick Start Cannabis Salve, Ointment, or Massage Oil** (pages 5–10) leftovers will have the greatest warming effect.

Quick Start Cooling Cannabis Poultice

leftover cannabis flower or trim material from the **Basic Quick Start Cannabis Salve, Ointment, or Massage Oil** Recipe (page 5)
1 bunch fresh mint leaves
1 tablespoon (15 ml) cold water
a few ice chips to cool the mix
a blender
clean wrapping gauze

Poultices have long been a part of traditional medicine across many cultures. Typically these preparations consist of ground or macerated herbs, clays, and resins that are applied directly to the skin. For example, some ancient texts from India reference fresh cannabis leaves applied directly to the skin as a poultice.

This cooling poultice contains cannabis and some common kitchen herbs. It also makes use of the leftover plant material from the **Basic Quick Start Cannabis Salve, Ointment, or Massage Oil** Recipe, which contains no warming spices.

1. Put the cannabis material, mint leaves, and water into the blender and blend until smooth. Add an ice chip and blend again briefly to cool the mixture down.
2. Apply this paste to the desired area and wrap with clean gauze. Apply additional ice packs or other moist cooling wraps as needed.

TIP: This recipe also makes a great forehead compress. Prepare the mixture as you would for a wrap, but instead apply to the forehead and temple area, then place a cold washcloth or compress over the area.

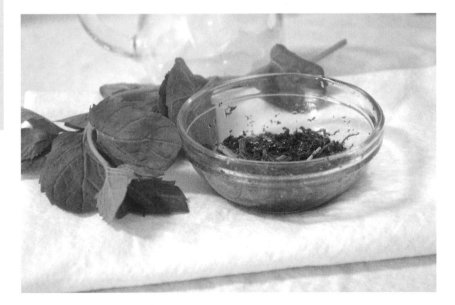

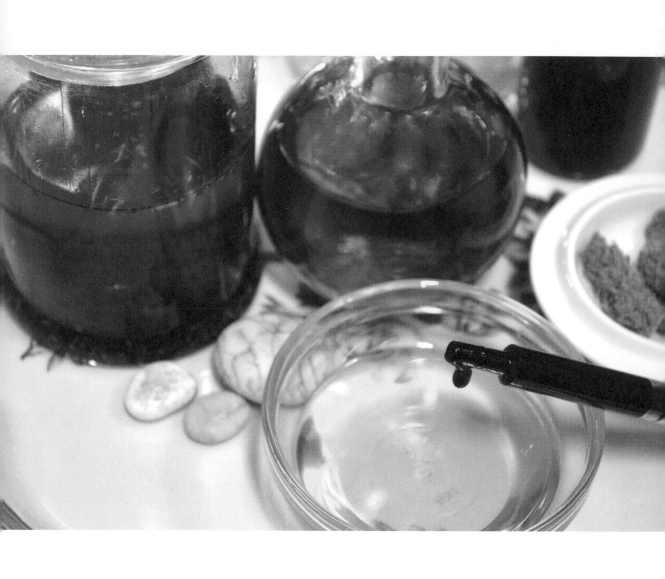

CHAPTER ONE: THE FOUNDATION—INGREDIENTS AND TECHNIQUES

In this chapter, you'll learn about the ingredients and techniques used to make the simplest to the most luxurious cannabis topical preparations.

I am a home herbalist, making my own external cannabis products to treat the sometimes unrelenting pain of autoimmune disease and to ameliorate side effects from the life-saving drugs and medical treatments I've had.

I've taught myself to make external cannabis preparations with ingredients that are free of artificial colors, flavors, fragrances, and preservatives. This makes these preparations as allergen-free and immune-system-friendly as possible. But, as always, consult your doctor for allergy information and diagnosis if you are in doubt about any of the ingredients listed.

Most external cannabis preparations will not cause any psychoactive effect and will provide local somatic relief only. However, contact with mucous membranes and ingesting preparations intended for topical use may cause psychoactive effects. For intensive pain relief—including psychoactive effects—external cannabis products may be combined with cannabis baths and vaporized or edible cannabis.

My cannabis spa recipes rely on the basic principles of kitchen chemistry you are probably already familiar with as a home chef. The recipes in this book are based on simple food-grade ingredient formulas, basic kitchen techniques, and for the most part easily obtainable ingredients. You will be able to learn the art of making cannabis spa and wellness products quickly, without the headaches of mistake batches.

The Small-Batch Philosophy

These are small-batch recipes. External cannabis products work better and are much fresher when made in small batches that are used quickly. You may double or triple any recipe, but for the purposes of the home chef who makes these recipes for only one or two people, small batches are the best way to minimize waste while having a fresh product on hand at all times.

In the Quick Start chapter, you have already learned how to make simple cannabis ointments combining just a few ingredients and cold processing. These Quick Start techniques are similar to those used in many of the following recipes in this book.

Most spa recipes in this book are perishable because they contain food-grade ingredients. You'll be creating small batches of cannabis spa products every few weeks, so they will need to be refrigerated in most cases. Lotions, creams, and other spa preparations made with whole plant constituents that contain moisture will break down if not held in cold temperatures or have an added chemical to prevent the action of the biosphere on the organic material.

Most shelf-stable spa products must contain preservatives to prevent microbial growth. I don't use preservatives and I do not recommend them. This is why the preservative-free recipes in this book rely on small batches, refrigeration, and quick use (within 30 days as a rule of thumb).

> TIP: Antioxidants like vitamin E and grapefruit seed extract are not preservatives and cannot prevent microbial growth.

Understanding Preservatives

I've written a lot about this on my site—why I personally do not use or make products that have artificial preservatives. We're told that these products are safe for consumption—and, in a sense, they do make health and beauty products safer for public consumption off of the shelf.

I stopped using preservatives after being told to do so by one of my physicians due to an autoimmune condition that was affecting my eyes. What I found out in the days following that encounter with my physician astounded me: many common artificial preservatives have noted immune system dysregulation side effects according to their own material safety data sheets.

I believe the problem with preservatives stems from the fact that they perform a function that is intended to defeat the action of the biosphere. Our biosphere naturally breaks down organic matter into decay and other natural end products—this is the final destination of everything organic. Maybe defiance of nature, in this case, isn't such a great idea after all. Do you really need this stuff in or on your body to feel good or look great?

You won't believe how fabulous it feels to use a fresh, preservative-free lotion or scrub right out of the fridge. This is so refreshing and simple you will say "ahhhhhh!" And fresh, simple ingredients are not only luxurious, they're good for you, too.

The Ingredients: Oils, Herbs, Resins, Water, Waxes, Weed, Oh My!

It's wise to assemble a kit in which you can organize all your spa-making supplies. Most supplies you will need can be found already in your own kitchen. There are a few you may need to obtain at a local Asian or ethnic grocery, natural grocer, or online. At the end of this book, you will find a resource guide that will help you obtain the more exotic ingredients used in some recipes.

Many of the ingredients in these recipes are common in Asian and Middle Eastern cuisine and wellness preparations. Cannabis is also native to this area, so it is not surprising that the first medicinal cannabis traditions using topical applications originated in Asia's herbal apothecary.

Cannabis has a wonderful synergy with the herbs and spices originating from this region of the world.

The following ingredients constitute the basic cannabis spa–making supply kit you'll need to start making all of the recipes in this book. Feel free to add to your kit as you discover new fragrances and herbs!

It's my hope that, along with discovering new ways to experience wellness and joy with cannabis, you'll also discover the pleasure of experiencing many other fragrances and herbs.

Base Fats High in Oleic Acid

The recipes in this book utilize base fats high in oleic acid, because oleic acid is the most effective in delivering cannabinoids transdermally compared to any other kind of fatty acid. Fats high in oleic acid also absorb best into the skin, leaving less to make the skin sticky or oily.

Olive oil that is fresh and cold pressed is best, and the more fresh and virgin the olive oil, the higher oleic acid content; this is what you need to penetrate deeply into the skin. Olive oil is also an excellent skin softener.

Sunflower oil is another oil high in oleic acid and is also an excellent emollient. I use this oil in many recipes where the greenish color of olive may not work well.

Mango seed butter is a softer seed butter, also high in oleic acid, that comes from the seed of the mango fruit. It absorbs well into the skin and is a great substitute for shea butter, which may cause sensitivity in those allergic to latex. Keep in mind that mango seed butter may not be appropriate for some people with nut allergies.

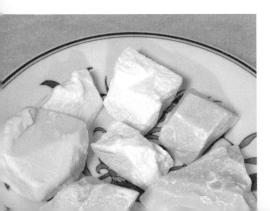

Cocoa butter comes from the cocoa bean and smells like a yummy chocolate bar! This butter is used in the Tropical Paradise Tanning Bar recipe. Cocoa butter is one of my all-time favorite oils for tanning because of its scent and beneficial emollient properties. It's also high in oleic acid.

Red palm oil is a bright reddish-orange oil pressed from the fruit of an African palm that is rich in carotenoids and antioxidants. Red palm oil has a buttery texture that is also high in oleic acid. For best results, select an organic palm oil that is food-grade with a deep color.

Tucuma and murumuru palm butters come from palm trees that provide a seed that produces a solid butter high in oleic acid. They are used in the lotion bar recipes. These butters have a slightly "soapy" fresh essence that work well with florals like rose.

Kokum butter is a hard seed butter from a fruit in the Mangosten family of trees. Its fatty acid profile—high in stearic acid and oleic acid—makes this butter suitable for making fresh cannabis lotion emulsions. Kokum butter also has a slightly "soapy" fresh essence that blends well with florals. Keep in mind that kokum may not be appropriate for some people with nut allergies.

Dry Ingredients

Sapindus mukorossi is also known as the soap nut or soapberry. The soapberry is a Himalayan treasure and is the centerpiece of the emulsion techniques you'll learn for creating cannabis baths, soaks, and washes. The soapberry emulsifies all oils and distributes them in the water, penetrating deeply into your skin instead of floating on the surface. The soapberry is also superior because it contains low-foaming saponins, which are a natural detergent. This makes it perfect for jet baths and other bath and soak applications. *Sapindus mukorossi* has been used for thousands of years in Ayurveda, a traditional medicine of India, for skin and hair health. It complements the cannabis herb perfectly.

Here in the West, people normally use soapberries for laundry purposes, as soapberries are commonly found in the laundry section of most natural food stores. Aside from their presence in the cannabis spa recipes in this book, soapberries make a superior all-around great household soap for those with allergies, skin conditions, or other special health needs. They are non-drying, anti-inflammatory, and antimicrobial. You don't need to wear gloves while cleaning your home with soapberries! This herbal water infused with saponins is both good for your skin and the environment.

At the end of this chapter, you will find recipes that are great for general cleaning and disinfecting and all use the authentic Sapindus mukorossi soapberry.

Pink Himalayan sea salt or any other sea salt—I like ancient salts the best for their fabulous mineral profile, which creates a very healing bathing experience.

Whole earth clays like sea clays, green clays, Moroccan red clays—all of these clays are rich in minerals and easy to find. Any good whole earth clay will work well with the mask and poultice spa recipes in this book.

Citrus peels fresh and dried—You'll need citrus peels to make the basic bath recipes and some of the bath salts. Some recipes call for blood orange peels, but you may substitute these with regular orange peels. Blood orange peels have the fragrance of orange, with a slight note of berry. They add a pink or reddish color to the recipes.

Spice mix—The recipes use an assortment of spices and herbs to impart fragrance and healing properties. Whole spices are recommended for best results, and examples include: cinnamon

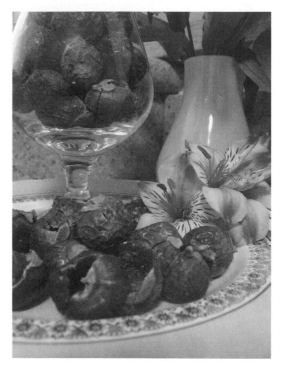

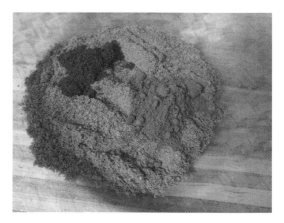

sticks, cardamom pods, cloves, star anise, turmeric root, black tea, white tea, roses, and ginger root.

Fresh flowers and herbs—Be sure to have some roses, citrus leaves and flowers, garden herbs, mints, lavender, and other fragrant herbs and flowers on hand!

Essential Oils

Pick your favorite! Luxury ingredients are used in some of the recipes here, such as floral attars, but you can use any of your favorite essential oils with these recipes, including jasmine, rose, ylang ylang, lavender, peppermint, rosemary, ginger, lemon, and henna flower.

Sunflower lecithin is an essential ingredient for creating the emulsions that become lotions, creams, and other preparations. It is free of GMO and industrial additives. I purchase sunflower lecithin in capsule form. The capsules can be broken open and the lecithin squeezed out. This is very convenient when measuring lecithin in the recipes because the capsules are already in 1 gram pre-measured sizes. *Do not* use dried sunflower lecithin in any of the recipes in this book; it will not emulsify properly. The lecithin needs to be very sticky and slightly waxy. Some brands are slightly more liquid than others—this is not a problem, as any "wet" sunflower lecithin will emulsify properly.

Waxes

Carnauba wax is a naturally occurring palm leaf wax. It makes a great vegetable substitute for beeswax in these recipes. Some of these recipes perform better with beeswax, as is noted in those recipes. Carnauba is quite hard and brittle and requires less material to contribute the same amount of solidification in recipes like the cannabis lotion bars. Use ½ to ⅔ as much carnauba as you would beeswax. My favorite use for carnauba wax is in the lip balm formulations to give them more staying power.

Beeswax is used in some cannabis topical products. It contributes a lovely fragrance profile you just can't get anywhere else. Beeswax is more pliable than carnauba, and it's my preferred wax for most of the recipes that require wax. If you have allergies, be aware that beeswax may contain some pollen and fungus, depending on the quality of its filtration.

Floral Waters, Hydrosols, and Aloe Vera

Floral waters, or "Hydrosols"—You can get these at an ethnic grocery, natural store, or online. They are a product of a process that uses steam distillation to extract the essential oils. They come in fragrances like rose, neroli, and mint. You'll see these most frequently available as "rose water," "orange flower water," "orris root water," and "mint water" in retail bottle packaging. These retail floral waters are normally used as flavorings for food and drink.

Floral waters are food-grade and should only contain citric acid in addition to distilled water. They should not contain any other preservatives. Floral waters require refrigeration after they are opened.

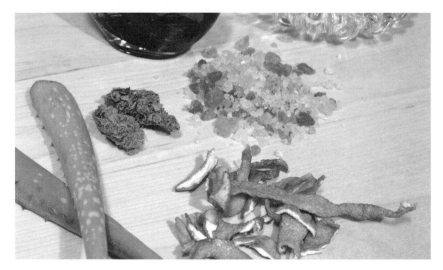

You can make your own essence water that performs functionally like the commercial hydrosols. Essence water is made through a process defined in chapter 5. Essence waters are not distilled, so they have a very short refrigeration life. They are best used within three days.

Aloe vera is used frequently in the recipes in this book. I almost exclusively use fresh aloe vera gel, harvested directly from fresh leaves. Aloe is a bit "chunky" when it is scraped fresh, but in these recipes the gel is blended smoothly in a blender before adding it to lotions or other preparations. Aloe vera gel contributes to the emulsification of lotions, baths, and other recipes while also providing skin-soothing and healing properties of its own.

Everything Else

Sanitizing products—My simple Soapberry Thieves recipe is great for sanitizing your counters and cooking equipment. Brewer's iodine is best for sanitizing containers. The potential for microbial contamination in spa products is as great, if not greater, than in food products, so you'll want to sanitize all containers and surfaces before starting your work.

Assorted glassware, glass bowls, a warming and cooking pan, and wooden utensils—Use these to make and store your cannabis spa products. My favorite glass for storing cannabis spa preparations is a dark violet glass, sold under various brand names like Miron and Violet Flame. This glass appears black and filters out all but a few essential colors in the light spectrum. This extends the life and freshness of the contents stored. Dark violet glass is the best option, in my experience, for keeping preservative-free preparations fresh and fully vital.

Cannabinoid-Containing Materials

Clean, finely ground cannabis flowers—These are a must-have ingredient. Even if you don't have access to concentrated cannabis products, you can make any of these recipes using cannabis flowers. Trim is not used in most of the recipes that follow this chapter; however, trim can be used with the bath recipes in chapter 3.

Full-Extract Cannabis Oil (also known as "Simpson Oil")— Popularized by cancer survivor Rick Simpson, this unique oil is fully decarboxylated and ready for use. No need to cook or heat.

Simpson Oil will stain your skin slightly green from the chlorophyll when used in a topical preparation, so you may not want to use it in preparations where you need to avoid staining skin or clothing. This is a whole food extract of cannabis made through an alcohol distillation process. The resulting oil contains all the original plant properties, including chlorophyll. Simpson Oil is best for topical applications that call for intensive medicinal benefits—chlorophyll stains and all!

Keif or Hashish—A raw, concentrated cannabis product, like ground flowers, that has not been decarboxylated. This is the best concentrated cannabis product for creating cannabis oils with little or no green coloration. Keif is fluffy and lighter, while hashish is sticky and heavier.

Working with Cannabis

Before you can begin making these products, you will need to create concentrated, fat-based cannabis preparation bases. This is important because the cannabinoids in cannabis are not water-soluble so they require fats or alcohol to dissolve properly.

The recipes in this book utilize decarboxylation, which is the same technique used to make cannabis food products. Decarboxylation is a chemical reaction that sheds carbon atoms from carbon chains when cannabinoids are heated to approximately 200–260 degrees Fahrenheit or 95–125 degrees Celsius for 30–120 minutes, depending on the end result you desire. If any of this sounds complicated, it isn't—basic cooking skills are all that are required to make really effective cannabis spa preparations.

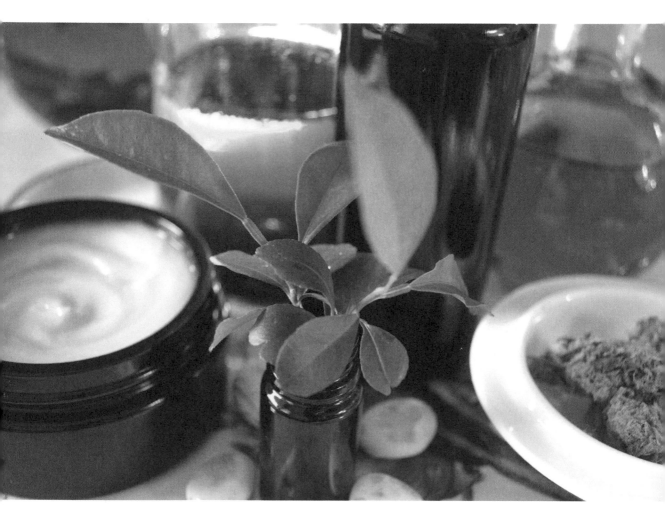

The "Does Everything" Cannabis Flower Foundation Oil

You will be making a fully decarboxylated cannabis oil in an oil base that is high in oleic acids. This "foundation oil" is called for in many recipes that follow in subsequent chapters. It is the foundation those recipes are built upon, alongside similar preparation methods found in the **Quick Start** recipes. These suggested foundation oils are more concentrated with cannabinoids and use the water and oil preparation method which is useful for eliminating some of the more pungent cannabis odors so that your other fragrances take center stage in the final spa preparation that you are making.

The only spa recipes in this book that don't use the "foundation oil" are the bath recipes, which use a different cannabis oil technique during the cooking process.

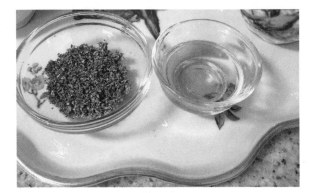 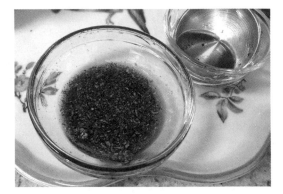

Water and oil preparation using a lidded pan on the stove, rice cooker, or slow cooker:

1 cup (240 ml) any of the high oleic acid oils or butters in this chapter
½ ounce (14 grams) or more finely ground cannabis flowers*
3 cups (720 ml) water

1. Pour the oil or butter and cannabis material into the pan or cooker along with 3 cups (720 ml) of water and stir.

2. If you are using a pan on the stove, set on low heat and simmer slowly with the lid on (do not boil) for 1 hour. I've let this heat as long as 2 hours, but I think the final fragrance of the oil is better between the 60 to 90-minute mark.

3. If you are using a rice cooker, set for a normal brown rice cooking cycle, which should take 30–45 minutes. After the cooking cycle is complete, allow this to remain on warm for 30 minutes.

4. If you are using a slow cooker, set on low and cook for 4 hours.

5. It may be necessary to add additional water for longer cooking times, but typically 3 cups (720 ml) of water will last the entire cooking cycle. Do not allow the oil to burn or "fry" the plant matter, as this will change the fragrance and composition of the essential oils.

6. Line a strainer with three layers of cheesecloth and strain. Squeeze the last of the liquid from the plant material and set aside the plant material for additional recipes.

7. After the oil and water have completely cooled and separated at room temperature, siphon the oil from the top using a syringe and transfer into the sterilized glass bottle or jar to be stored in a cool, dark place or in the refrigerator. It's important to ensure that water is not transferred to the sterile oil jar, so leave a thin oil slick on top of the water after siphoning for the storage jar, then siphon that up separately. Use it immediately in a lotion recipe, or just straight from the syringe, to soothe your skin immediately!

---

* Strains rich in cannabinoids work the best. Select your favorite strain with the qualities that appeal to you the most. Double the amount for strains lower in cannabinoids.

Keif or Hashish Foundation Oil

Keif is my favorite form of raw cannabis when making foundation oil because of its versatility. Keif will produce the least amount of pungent cannabis fragrance in the final oil when prepared in the stove top method described here.

1 cup (240 ml) any of the high oleic acid oils or butters in this chapter
6–10 grams or more keif or hashish
2 cups (480 ml) water

Keif or hashish is more powerful than the ground cannabis flower because they contain more cannabinoids and less plant material.

The basic recipe calls for 6 grams of keif or hashish. You may use more or less, but in my test kitchen, 6 grams was the most effective for making suitably cannabinoid-rich topical products.

The other advantage in using keif or hashish is that the final foundation oil product has less green color than those made with cannabis flowers. The **Tropical Tanning Bar**, for example, calls for blonde keif; the more blonde or lightly colored your concentrated cannabis product, the lighter the foundation oil will be.

Preparation using a lidded pan on the stove:

1. Pour the oil or butter and cannabis material into the pan along with 2 cups (480 ml) of water and stir.
2. Set on low heat and allow this to simmer slowly with the lid on (do not boil) for 1 hour. I've let this heat as long as 2 hours, but I think the final fragrance of the oil is better between the 60 to 90-minute mark.
3. It may be necessary to add additional water for longer cooking times, but typically 2 cups (480 ml) of water will last the entire cooking cycle. Do not allow the oil to burn or "fry" the plant matter, as this will change the fragrance and composition of the essential oils.
4. Line a strainer with three layers of cheesecloth and strain. Squeeze the last of the liquid from the plant material—there probably won't be much since you are working with keif or hashish.
5. After the oil and water have completely cooled and separated at room temperature, siphon the oil from the top using a syringe and transfer into the sterilized glass bottle or jar to be stored in a cool, dark place or in the refrigerator. It's important to ensure that water is not transferred to the sterile oil jar, so leave a thin oil slick on top of the water after siphoning for the storage jar and siphon that up separately. Use it immediately in a lotion recipe, or just straight from the syringe, to soothe your skin immediately!

Full–Extract Cannabis Oil ("Simpson Oil" or RSO) Foundation Oil

6–10 grams or more full-extract cannabis oil
1 cup (240 ml) any of the high oleic acid oils or butters in this chapter

If you use full-extract cannabis oil (otherwise known as "Simpson Oil" or RSO), making a foundation oil for use with these recipes is very simple and requires only warming heat. Simpson Oil is fully decarboxylated and it also contains a significant amount of chlorophyll, which may impart a slight green tint to your skin. This is why this oil is best used in recovery and healing applications, as in the traditional **Kaneh Bosem** recipe.

1. Fully dissolve the tar-like full-extract cannabis oil into the base oil using a gentle warm heat.
2. Transfer oil mixture to a clean, sterile glass jar. Store in a cool, dark place or in the refrigerator.

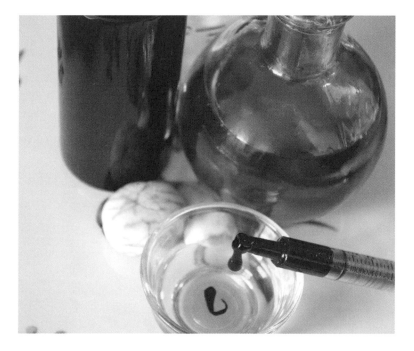

The Secret of Ancients

Kaneh Bosem Anointing Oil for the Healing of the Nations

In 1936, as cannabis and hemp were about to become illegal for the first time in the United States, a Polish anthropologist who studied Judaic culture, Sula Benet, suggested that kaneh bosem—mentioned throughout the Bible—was not reed calamus as most scholars believe, but rather the fragrant cannabis-hemp reed. This debate continues even today.

Did the holy anointing oil prescribed by G-d for the priests in the Old Testament, and used generously to heal the sick by Jesus in the New Testament, contain cannabis? I don't know the answer to this question, but I suspect that it did.

The *cannabis var. indica* plant, a highly psychoactive and fragrant strain, is native to central Asia. Sula Benet's interpretation makes sense in light of the fragrance and other qualities described in the original holy texts. The fragrance profile of *cannabis var. indica* is unique because its flowers have such a wide range of powerful fragrances, including fruits, spices, coffee, vanilla, lavender, citrus peels, and more.

For me, the proof lies in the effectiveness of the healing qualities of the formulation as described in the holy texts. **Kaneh Bosem Healing Oil** is one of my go-to oils when my joint pain levels are at their worst. There is a synergy between cannabis and the other essential oils in this preparation that is, in my opinion, unparalleled for pain relief.

The combination of herbs in this ancient recipe creates a wellness formula that is very effective, yet simple enough to make at home.

> **22** Moreover the Lord spake unto Moses, saying, **23** Take thou also unto thee principal spices, of pure myrrh five hundred shekels, and of sweet cinnamon half so much, even two hundred and fifty shekels, and of *kaneh bosem two hundred and fifty shekels, **24** And of cassia five hundred shekels, after the shekel of the sanctuary, and of oil olive an hin: **25** And thou shalt make it an oil of holy ointment, an ointment compound after the art of the apothecary: it shall be an holy anointing oil."
>
> Exodus 30: 22-25 KJV
> *calamus mistranslation
> — Sula Benet

The Herbs

Cassia and Cinnamon Bark Essential Oils—The kaneh bosem anointing oil recipe calls for two fragrant trees that produce what is commonly known today as cinnamon. Most cinnamon available on the grocery shelves is in fact cassia cinnamon, a less expensive variety.

True Ceylon cinnamon (Cinnamomum verum **or** Cinnamomum zeylanicum) is a rare variety, with a different fragrance than that of cassia, which is slightly more floral or sweet. Both of these cinnamon essential oils are used together in this recipe to create a warming and soothing sensation that increases circulation in painful joints and muscles.

Myrrh is an ancient tree resin from the Middle East that is used in fragrances, incense, and mouthwash. It has anti-inflammatory and antimicrobial properties. It also has a very earthy scent that pairs well with cannabis. This recipe calls for myrrh essential oil in addition to cinnamon and cassia oils.

Olive oil was the most common oil available in biblical times and is also very high in oleic acid. And as we know, oleic acid is best for aiding in the absorption of cannabinoids from external preparations.

Kaneh bosem or cannabis (It's likely no mistake that those names sound alike!) My favorite way to make **Kaneh Bosem Healing Oil** is with **Full-Extract Cannabis Oil**, known as "Simpson Oil" or RSO. It's the best pain relief recipe here! But for those who may not have access to "Simpson Oil" (RSO), this recipe can be made with another Cannabis Foundation Oil from this chapter.

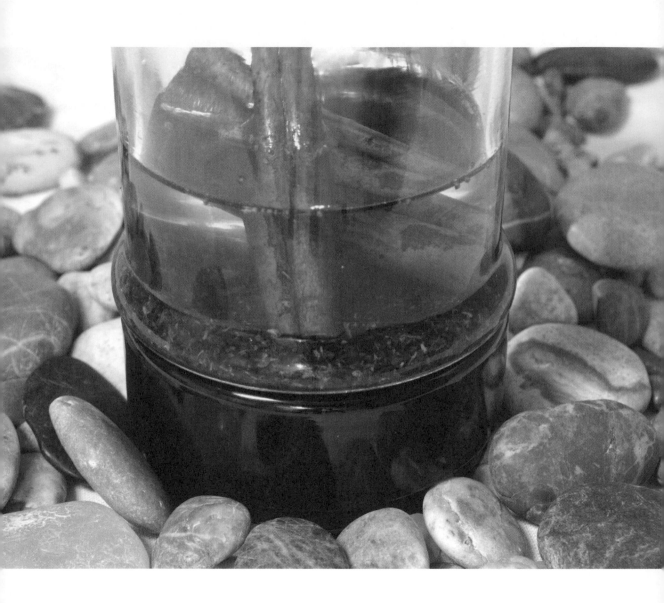

Kaneh Bosem Healing Oil

½ cup (120 ml) cold-pressed, virgin olive oil

15 drops myrrh essential oil

3 drops common cassia cinnamon oil

3 drops True Ceylon cinnamon essential oil (*Cinnamomum verum* or *Cinnamomum zeylanicum*)

½ cup (120 ml) **Cannabis Foundation Oil** (page 36), made with olive oil*

---

* **The Full-Extract Cannabis Oil** or "Simpson Oil" recipe from this chapter produces the best results.

whole, cured, and very dry cannabis flowers, vape tailings, or trim

myrrh resin

cinnamon sticks from one or more species of cinnamon

olive oil

1. Thoroughly combine all ingredients and store in the refrigerator for 2 or more hours.
2. This oil will partially solidify into a semi-soft ointment, but will still be easy to stir. Stir this ointment thoroughly before use.

This healing oil may be used right from the jar, or you can use it to prepare convenient lotion bars and fluffy refrigerated cold creams.

When this oil is used directly, without further dilution in bars or lotions, it is extremely concentrated with essential oils and cannabinoids, so a small amount goes a long way. It's also more effective when used with hot, moist towel wraps or after a hot shower or bath.

Aged Kaneh Bosem Healing Oil

In the Quick Start chapter, you've learned how to make **Herbal Spa Oil Jars** with vape tailings, which are infused with herbs and then aged for a few months. By preparing authentic **Kaneh Bosem Healing Oil** in this manner, you will produce an exquisite oil by using the same aging process with fresh, dried herbs and resins.

1. Fill a clean and sterile glass jar loosely with equal amounts of whole cannabis flowers, myrrh resin, and cinnamon sticks.
2. Pour olive oil over the dry ingredients until they are covered, leaving a small space at the top.
3. Close tightly and store in a cool, dark place. Age for 6 or more months for the best results.
4. Refresh the levels of olive oil as you use this **Kaneh Bosem Healing Oil**.

I'm a Soapberry Evangelist, and You Should Be, Too!

You've already read about the soapberry (*Sapindus mukorossi*) earlier in this chapter, and all the various ways it can be used for sanitizing your working area, in addition to the emulsification techniques used in recipes that will follow in subsequent chapters.

Soapberries can perform any job—and quite well, I might add—that any commercially prepared soap, shampoo, detergent, or cleaner can tackle. If you want to avoid preservatives, it is important to remember that many shelf-stable liquid soaps and cleansers, regardless of the organic labeling, may contain a preservative to prevent spoilage. Soapberries are dried first and activated with water later, so they never require a preservative, only refrigeration subsequent to activation.

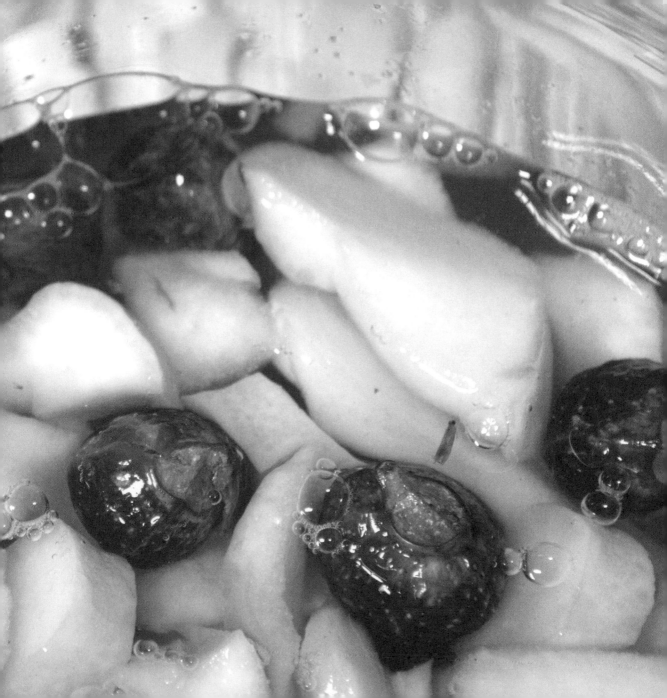

Basic Soapberry Liquid for Hair and Skin

Skin sensitivities and allergies? This soapberry preparation is simple to make and very refreshing. Soapberry liquid is naturally low-foaming, which may take some adjustment if you are fond of the mountains of foam that many commercial shampoos and soaps produce on contact with water. Strained through a muslin or coffee filter, this soapberry liquid works great in a foam dispenser bottle and will actually foam quite nicely.

My favorite method for mountains of silky soapberry foam uses a manual milk foamer, such as those used to foam milk for espresso. They're inexpensive and easy to use in the shower or bath. Just fill the bottom of the foamer with a little concentrated soapberry soap liquid, then plunge the foamer vigorously to create lots of thick soap foam!

Soapberries have an earthy, cooked pineapple or vinegar fragrance. This recipe optionally adds a few citrus peels to the soapberry liquid (lemon or orange), along with a drop or two of essential oil.

50 *Sapindus Mukorossi* soapberries, seeded and split in half
a few citrus peels, dried or fresh, optional
3 cups (720 ml) water
any essential oil of your choice, optional

1. Briefly rinse the dry soapberries in a strainer and add to the bowl. Then add a few citrus peels and cannabis, if you choose.
2. Boil the water and pour it over the dry ingredients in the bowl. Cover and allow this to sit overnight or 6–8 hours.
3. Put the mixture on the stove and heat on medium for 15 minutes. Using a masher, mash/pound the soapberry mixture to release the saponin liquid; the soapberries should now be plump from water absorption. Set aside mixture to cool for 2 or more hours.
4. Use a strainer or cloth bag to strain the mixture, squeezing out as much liquid as possible, and set the leftovers aside.
5. If you plan to use the liquid in a soap pump, prepare a muslin cloth or coffee filter to use in your strainer and pour the liquid through the strainer to remove excess plant material. Add essential oils if you prefer; 2 or more drops of any essential oil are best if you want to add fragrance to this gentle cleanser.

At this point, you have a very concentrated soap liquid that is ready to be bottled. Keep this cleanser refrigerated when not in use. Don't panic if you forget it for a couple of days! The cleanser won't go bad that quickly, but it does require extended refrigeration to maintain its freshness.

TIP: Some people like to use cannabis in this recipe for relief from various skin conditions. Doing this is easy, just add 1 gram of finely ground cannabis flowers.

TIP: Combine the leftover soapberry mixture with a bowl or basin of warm water. Agitate and strain, and use this secondary soap liquid right away to wash your hair or body!

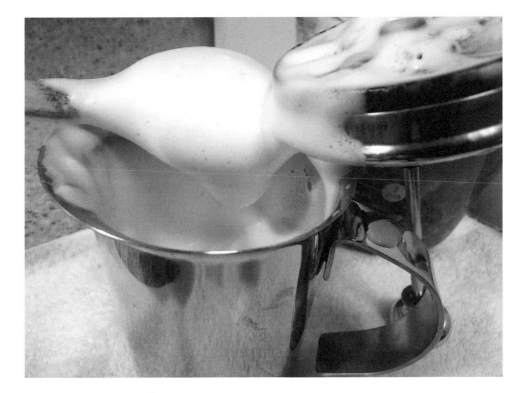

Cannabis Oil Scalp Treatment for Itchy Scalp

Use this recipe as a scalp treatment for an irritated or itchy scalp by using 1 tablespoon (15 ml) of **Cannabis Foundation Oil**. This treatment should only be used on the scalp before washing hair and not after, as the cannabis oils are too sticky to serve as a hair conditioner.

Massage a small amount into your scalp—but not your hair—and allow this to remain for 30 minutes before washing with the soapberry concentrate.

1. Melt all of the oils together until warm, then add the essential oils as desired.
2. Pour into a glass bottle or container. Shake well. This oil can be stored in cool, dark place for up to 3 months.

2 tablespoons (30 milliliters) hemp seed oil
2 tablespoons (30 milliliters) olive oil
1 tablespoon (15 milliliters) **Cannabis Foundation Oil** (page 36)
5 drops lavender essential oil
2 drops blue chamomile essential oil

Soapberries at Home

Other Uses for Soapberries

In the Dishwasher or Hand Washing Dishes
Soapberries are great for soaking, washing dishes, and they work in the dishwasher, too! Add a few to your dish pan or the utensil holder in your dishwasher to aid in the washing process.
Laundry
Throw 4–5 shelled soapberries in a muslin bag and toss in the washer. To whiten laundry, add oxygen "bleach." Prepare stains before laundering using a natural orange oil stain treatment.

If you'd like an effective, healthy, and environmentally friendly way to clean up and disinfect, soapberries are excellent for laundry, dishwashers, and as a general home cleanser. Soapberries are antimicrobial and do a great job on dirt and odors without exposing you or your family to preservatives or harmful chemicals. For really greasy stains or cleaning jobs, you can use an orange-based degreaser before washing with soapberries.

Soapberry Thieves

This recipe is based on a very popular article from hempista.com about the use of essential oils as a disinfectant and how some forward-looking modern hospitals have adopted essential oil technology to combat the spread of infection. This disinfectant recipe is further based on a historical recipe reputed to be from the Middle Ages, called Four Thieves Vinegar.

Legend has it that a band of thieves were able to rob the dead during the Black Plague in Europe while not infecting themselves by using a vinegar that was steeped in certain herbs. At some point, they were finally caught and, in a bargain made to spare their lives, they revealed the recipe that enabled their profitable exploits amongst the dead. The recipe handed down since that time consists of essential oils now known to have antimicrobial and antiviral properties, specifically the pungent and fragrant herbs available during that time in Europe, such as lavender, thyme, citrus, and rosemary.

It's easy to re-create this healthy disinfectant using a few drops of essential oils, hot water, and soapberries!

5 or more whole, dried *Sapindus Mukorossi* soapberries, broken into 2 or more pieces essential oils—lavender, thyme, lemon, and rosemary

1. Run scalding water in a bucket over the dried soapberries and add 2 or more drops of each essential oil.
2. Agitate until sudsy.

The soapberries may be removed later and used in another batch of disinfectant so don't throw them out! They are usually good for 3–4 average-sized buckets of disinfecting cleanser.

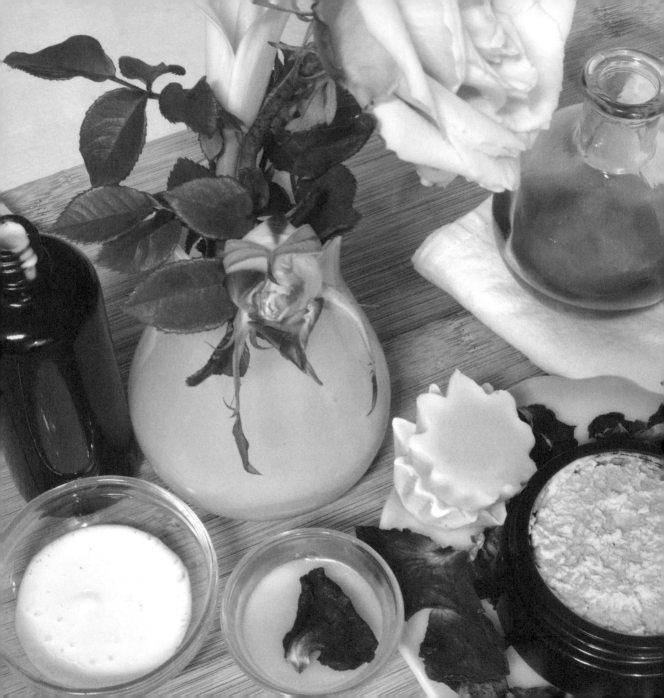

CHAPTER TWO: LOTIONS, CREAMS, AND SCRUBS

Cannabis lotion, creams, and scrubs are some of the best ways to enjoy the healing and beauty benefits of externally applied cannabis without experiencing psychoactive side effects.

All these recipes are fully decarboxylated and rich in oleic acids, which is key in effectively delivering cannabinoids transdermally. All ingredients listed here are fully explained in chapter 1 and can be purchased using the resource guide at the end of the book. In my personal experience, most ingredients are readily available locally.

Cannabis Lotion Bars

Lotion bars are a lush treat that are easy to make and very portable! If this is your first time making lotions or creams, starting with these lotion bars is a foolproof way to begin and is also quite satisfying.

Lotion bars are best when refrigerated, but because they don't contain water, they are actually shelf-stable for about 3 months. The fats, oils, and waxes can become "grainy" in natural spa preparations like lotion bars when preparations are left to cool completely at room temperature, so prompt cooling by refrigeration ensures that these spa creations are rich and creamy. Be sure to follow the recipe instructions precisely, as they call for an initial cooling period at room temperature before refrigeration. This allows the preparation to solidify properly.

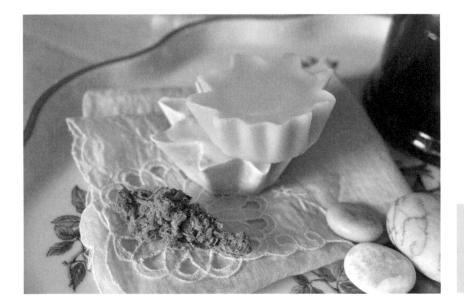

TIP: Silicon muffin molds work well when making lotion bars if you don't have any soap or candy molds.

Warming Herbs Recovery Bar

½ cup (120 milliliters) mango seed butter

½ cup (120 milliliters) tucuma or murumuru butter

3 tablespoons (45 milliliters) beeswax

1 teaspoon (2 grams) cayenne pepper powder

¼ cup (60 milliliters) **Cannabis Foundation Oil** (page 36)

10 drops ginger essential oil

3 drops any cinnamon essential oil

This recipe uses warming herbs, along with fats high in oleic acid, to prepare solid warming bars great for use on sore muscles (or at any time). I've found these bars to be effective for sciatica pain. I've also received positive reports from others about their effectiveness in reducing neuropathic pain.

This recipe contains cayenne pepper and should not be used near the eyes or other mucous membranes.

Makes three or four small bars

1. Melt the butters and wax together with the cayenne pepper powder. Add the cannabis oil and essential oils after the mixture has melted, and stir. Pour into molds immediately.

2. Allow this to cool on the counter for 15 minutes then transfer immediately to the refrigerator for 2 or more hours. This produces solid bars that are easily popped away from the mold.

Store wrapped in parchment paper in the refrigerator for up to 6 months. These bars are shelf stable for about 3 months.

Thai Stick Lemongrass Scrub Bar

Superb for scrubbing scaly irritated skin, this lotion bar brings together the great qualities of the Thai Stick Lemongrass Lotion recipe in a bar form by using coarse demerara sugar crystals for a great exfoliating treatment that's healing, soothing, and sweet—just like the cannabis strain it's named after.

Makes three or four small bars

1. Melt the butters and wax together. Add the cannabis and lemongrass oil to the melted mixture.
2. Add the sugar and stir briskly, then pour immediately into molds.
3. Allow this to cool on the counter for 15 minutes, then transfer immediately to the refrigerator for 2 or more hours. This produces solid bars that are easily popped away from the mold.

The bottom side of the bar will have a concentration of sugar crystals and cannabis herb after it hardens. Use this side of the bar for scrubbing. You can store these bars wrapped in baking parchment in the refrigerator for up to 6 months. These bars are stable at room temperature for about 3 months.

½ cup (120 milliliters) mango seed butter

½ cup (120 milliliters) tucuma or murumuru butter

1 tablespoon (15 milliliters) beeswax or carnauba wax

1 tbsp (2g) ground cannabis leaf or flower

10 drops lemongrass essential oil

2 tablespoons (25 grams) coarse demerara sugar crystals

Cannabis Beauty Body Bar

½ cup (120 milliliters) mango seed butter

½ cup (120 milliliters) tucuma or murumuru butter

3 tablespoons (45 milliliters) beeswax

¼ cup (60 milliliters) **Cannabis Foundation Oil** (page 36)

5 drops jasmine essential oil

2 drops rose essential oil

1 drop True Ceylon cinnamon essential oil (*Cinnamomum verum* or *Cinnamomum zeylanicum*)

2 drops neroli or orange blossom essential oil

Looking for a really lush and sensual beauty body bar that smells divine? These bars are great for moisturizing all over after a shower or bath. They have a classic floral fragrance based on natural jasmine and other essential oils.

Makes three or four small bars

1. Melt the butters and wax together, add the cannabis oil and essential oils after the mixture has melted and stir. Pour into molds immediately.

2. Allow this to cool on the counter for 15 minutes, then transfer immediately to the refrigerator for 2 or more hours. This produces solid bars that are easily popped away from the mold.

Store these bars wrapped in parchment paper in the refrigerator for up to 6 months. These bars are shelf stable for about 3 months.

Ancient Healer Kaneh Bosem Lotion Bars

One of my favorite ways to enjoy the healing benefits of the ancient kaneh bosem medicine is in a lotion bar. Using the traditional ancient kaneh bosem formula as the base, this recipe adds additional herbal medicine ingredients to soothe your aches and pains, along with a natural fragrance profile that I hope will transport you back in time to an ancient healing spa. This recipe includes fossilized amber essential oil, black pepper essential oil, boswellia resin, and frankincense essential oil.

Makes three or four small bars

1. Melt the butters, oil, and boswellia resin together on low heat until all but the gum of the resin (which is not oil soluble) remains at the bottom. It will have a sand-like consistency. Strain the oil until it is clear.
2. Melt the beeswax in the oil using low heat, then add the essential oils.
3. Pour the warm oil into the molds, and allow it to cool on the counter for 15 minutes.
4. Transfer immediately to the refrigerator for 2 or more hours. This produces solid bars that are easily popped away from the mold.

Store wrapped in parchment paper in the refrigerator for up to 6 months. These bars are shelf stable at room temperature for about 3 months.

¼ cup (60 milliliters) mango seed butter

⅓ cup (78 milliliters) kokum butter

½ cup (120 milliliters) **Kaneh Bosem Healing Oil** (page 40)

2 teaspoons (10 grams) powdered or ground boswellia resin

3 tablespoons (45 milliliters) beeswax

3 drops black pepper essential oil

5 drops frankincense essential oil

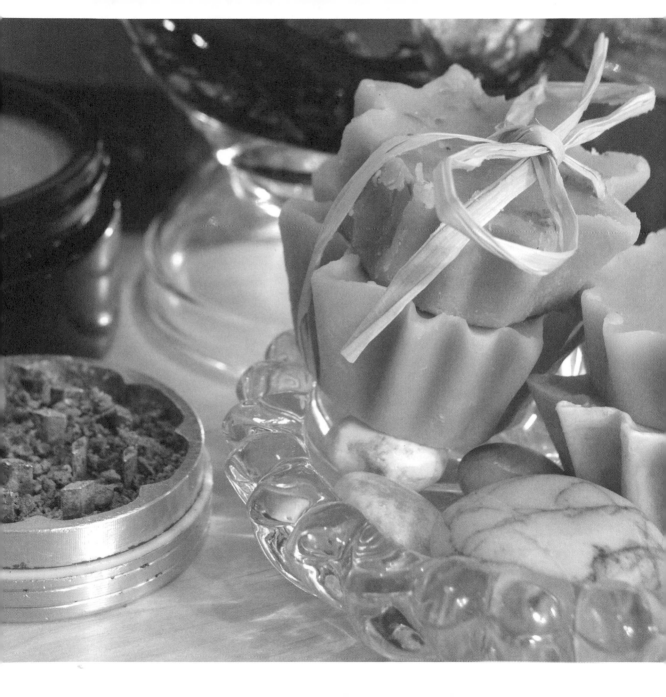

Paradise Tanning Lotion Bars

Cannabis has many known anticancer properties, which makes it a great choice for sun-drenched skin treatment. There are two formulas to suit your tanning needs: **The Tropical Paradise** (humid tanning) and **The Desert Paradise** (dry tanning) formulas. Both formulas use exotic essential oils and seed butters, high in oleic acid, along with cannabis—all of which will deliver paradise to your skin!

These tanning lotion bars are deeply moisturizing and great for use after sun exposure, too. Please note that these bars do not contain any SPF-rated sunscreen and are not intended to be used for that purpose.

The Desert Paradise Tanning Lotion Bar

Based on the fragrance of desert florals, resins, and dry minerals, this tanning lotion bar features henna flower attar, carnation flower essential oil, and a citrus-like frankincense essential oil, which creates a deep, ancient desert floral fragrance.

Makes three or four small bars

½ cup (120 milliliters) mango seed butter
½ cup (120 milliliters) kokum butter
2 tablespoons or (30 milliliters) beeswax
¼ cup (60 milliliters) **Cannabis Foundation Oil** (page 36)
10 drops frankincense essential oil
5 drops henna flower attar
5 drops carnation flower essential oil

1. Melt the butters and wax together. Add the cannabis oil and combine thoroughly with the essential oils.
2. Pour into molds and allow this to cool on the counter for 15 minutes.
3. Transfer immediately to the refrigerator for 2 or more hours. This produces solid bars that are easily popped away from the mold.

Store these bars wrapped in parchment paper in the refrigerator for up to 6 months. These bars are shelf stable at room temperature for about 3 months.

The Tropical Paradise Tanning Lotion Bar

¾ cup (180 milliliters) cold-pressed cocoa butter

1 tablespoon (15 milliliters) red palm oil

3 tablespoons (45 milliliters) beeswax

¼ cup (60 milliliters) **Cannabis Foundation Oil** (page 36)*

2 drops ylang ylang essential oil

3 drops tuberose essential oil

3 drops jasmine essential oil

This bar incorporates tuberose essential oil and red palm fruit butter, which gives it a golden color when used exclusively in a recipe with blonde keif or hashish. Ground cannabis flower will lend a green cast to this lotion bar. Either way, this bar will apply a beautiful sheer golden color to the skin due to the presence of red palm fruit butter.

Makes three or four small bars

1. Melt the cocoa butter, palm oil, and beeswax together. Add the cannabis oil and combine thoroughly with the essential oils.
2. Pour into molds and allow this to cool on the counter for 15 minutes.
3. Transfer immediately to the refrigerator for 2 or more hours. This produces solid bars that are easily popped away from the mold.

Store these bars wrapped in parchment paper in the refrigerator for up to 6 months. These bars are shelf stable at room temperature for about 3 months.

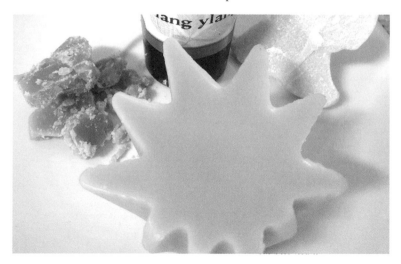

Apothecary Cannabis Rose Lotion Bar

These bars have an amazing ability to maintain their fragrance, even when they are left in the open air, as I have happened to do many times. Nevertheless, if you want to maintain the best fragrance, store these bars wrapped in parchment baking paper or bags.

Makes three or four small bars

1. Melt the butters and wax together, then add the cannabis oil and essential oils after the mixture has melted and stir. Pour into molds immediately.
2. Allow this to cool on the counter for 15 minutes, then transfer immediately to the refrigerator for 2 or more hours. This produces solid bars that are easily popped away from the mold.

Store these bars wrapped in parchment paper in the refrigerator for up to 6 months. These bars are shelf stable for about 3 months.

½ cup (120 milliliters) mango seed butter

½ cup (120 milliliters) kokum butter

3 tablespoons (45 milliliters) beeswax

¼ cup (60 milliliters) **Cannabis Foundation Oil** (page 36)

2 drops True Ceylon cinnamon essential oil (*Cinnamomum verum* or *Cinnamomum zeylanicum*)

5 drops rose or geranium rose essential oil

Apothecary Cannabis Rose Ancient Salt Scrub Bar

½ cup (120 milliliters) mango seed butter

½ cup (120 milliliters) tucuma or murumuru butter

1 tablespoon (15 milliliters) beeswax

leftover ground flower material from making the **Cannabis Foundation Oil** (page 36)

¼ cup (60 grams) ancient sea salt or Himalayan salt, fine to semi-coarse grind

1 drop True Ceylon cinnamon essential oil (*Cinnamomum verum* or *Cinnamomum zeylanicum*)

5 drops rose or geranium rose essential oil

3 drops essential lemon oil

This lively exfoliating scrub will take your tired and sallow skin from sad to fabulous! This scrub is fantastic for use prior to taking one of the cannabis baths from chapter 3.

Makes three or four small bars

1. Gently melt the butters and beeswax together. Stir in the cannabis, salt, and essential oils as the last step before pouring into molds.
2. Cool on the counter until almost hard, and then place in the refrigerator until the bars are hard enough to remove from the molds.

The salt and cannabis herbs will collect on the bottom of the bars while they are cooling, which creates a perfect scrub side! Store unused bars in the refrigerator up to 6 months. This bar will keep well at room temperature for 3 months.

Chocolate and Roses Lip Balm

Meet your new favorite lip balm! Valentine's Day is every day when you wear this tasty and very kissable cannabis lip balm. This recipe makes a solid balm that can be poured into a lip balm dispenser or into a small cosmetic lip gloss pot.

1. Melt the butter and wax. Add the cannabis oil, and cinnamon oil, and rose oil, stir, then pour into a container.
2. Finish by letting the preparation cool in the refrigerator for 2 or more hours.

This lip balm has a shelf life of roughly 2 months if carried in your purse or pocket frequently. Otherwise, when stored in a cool, dark place it should last for up to 3 months.

2 tablespoons (30 milliliters) cold-pressed and raw cacao butter

1 tablespoon (15 milliliters) carnauba wax or beeswax

2 tablespoons (30 milliliters) **Cannabis Foundation Oil*** (page 36)

1 drop True Ceylon cinnamon essential oil (*Cinnamomum verum* or *Cinnamomum zeylanicum*)

2 drops rose essential oil (don't substitute for best results)

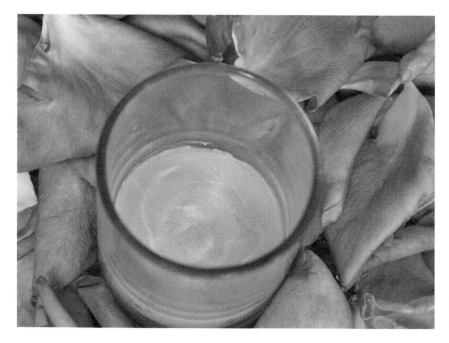

* Made with sunflower oil for the best results.

The Apothecary Cannabis Rose Recipes

Apothecary Rose, also known as *rose gallica* and Medieval Rose, is a small-medium ancient heirloom rose with a strong fragrance and color that varies from dark red to pink. This rose is a favorite for teas, herbal medicine, and beauty. It's closely related to the Damascus rose and other varieties of rose used in commercial oil and hydrosol production.

These cannabis rose recipes are based on the Apothecary Rose, which is known for its skin emollient and wrinkle-minimizing properties. These recipes rely on essential rose oils, fats, and hydrosols for their unique properties and fragrance.

When working with cannabis oils, it's important to round out the sharp, herbal scent of cannabis with other fragrances so the preparations are not overpowered by the scent of cannabis. Cannabis scents should play nicely with all the other scents; cannabis oils need not leave you smelling like your favorite cannabis dispensary! The Apothecary Cannabis Rose recipes, like some of the other recipes, achieve this effect with the addition of True Ceylon cinnamon oil. This allows the sharper notes of the cannabis flower to take a step back, revealing a gorgeous rose fragrance that is natural and not overpowering. Ceylon cinnamon has an almost fruity floral quality that sets it apart from the more common cassia variety of cinnamon. This plays extraordinarily well with the other flowers in these recipes.

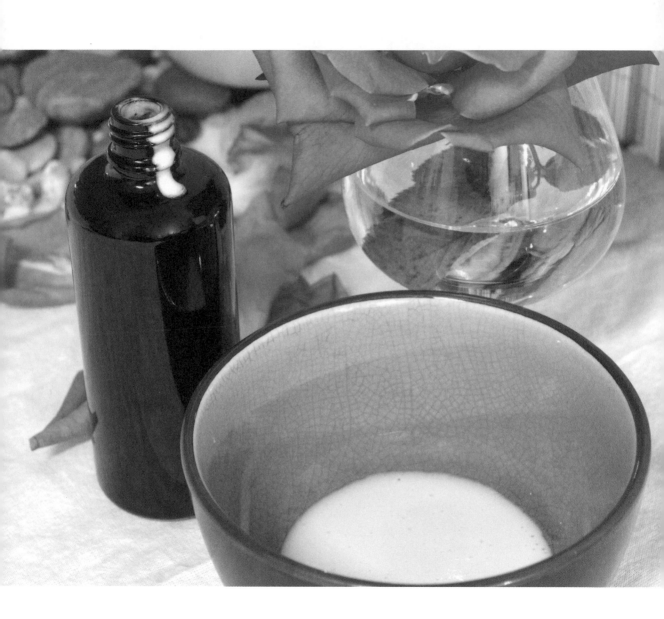

Making Creams and Lotions

Creams and lotions contain enough water when exposed to normal shelf storage conditions that they become hotbeds of microbial activity if they don't contain preservatives. For this reason, all off-the-shelf commercial cream and lotion products, organic or not, will contain preservatives.

As explained in chapter 1, preservatives may be avoided by creating small batches while keeping the product in refrigeration and by using the product within one month. This small batch philosophy applies to all lotion recipes made with high-quality food-grade ingredients.

Proper emulsification is another requirement for successful batches of lotions and creams. Emulsification guarantees that the moisturizing elements will not separate from the oils. There are two critical principles for proper emulsification:

1. All ingredients must be at the same temperature before mixing, typically around 140 degrees Fahrenheit (60 degrees Celsius). Ingredients are first heated to 175 degrees Fahrenheit (80 degrees Celsius), but never greater than 200 degrees Fahrenheit (93 degrees Celsius), and then allowed to cool briefly to the more optimal temperature before combining to create the emulsion.
2. An emulsifying agent must be present in the mixture. In these recipes, sunflower lecithin and aloe vera are the emulsifiers of choice.

By bringing all ingredients to the same temperature in a liquid state, along with an emulsifying agent, the resulting mixture produces luxurious cannabis lotions and creams. However, like the lotion bars and other spa potions containing a variety of solid and liquid fats, oils, and waxes, sometimes an undesirable "grainy" texture will result if the preparation is allowed to cool completely at room temperature. Be sure to follow the recipe instructions precisely, which will call for an initial cooling period at room temperature before placing the preparation in the refrigerator to set completely.

Emergency rescue for lotions and creams that don't come out right the first time:
Making lotions and creams isn't hard, but sometimes it's not as forgiving as other types of spa preparations. If your lotion or cream isn't to your liking, it's easy to reset the preparation by putting the entire lotion or cream back into a pan and heating to 175 degrees Fahrenheit (80 degrees Celsius), thereby melting and re-sanitizing the emulsion, and then whipping and cooling using the original recipe steps.

Apothecary Cannabis Rose Milk

A milky and quick absorbing lotion that will leave the slightest scent of roses, Apothecary Cannabis Rose Milk makes a great everyday moisturizer for the face or hands.

1. In a blender, combine rose water, lemon juice, and aloe vera gel for a few seconds until thoroughly smooth. Pour into a pan on the stove and heat to 175 degrees Fahrenheit (80 degrees Celsius).
2. Melt the mango seed butter, sunflower lecithin, and cannabis oil in a separate pan on the stove. Heat this mixture to 175 degrees Fahrenheit (80 degrees Celsius).

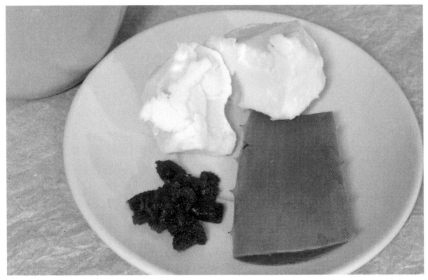

Clockwise from bottom: sunflower lecithin, mango seed butter, fresh aloe vera leaf

½ cup (120 milliliters)
distilled rose water

½ teaspoon (2 milliliters)
lemon juice

¼ cup (60 milliliters) aloe
vera gel, scraped from
the leaf

2 tablespoons
(30 milliliters) mango
seed butter

½ teaspoon (2.5 grams)
sunflower lecithin

¼ cup (60 milliliters)
**Cannabis Foundation
Oil*** (page 36)

1 drop True Ceylon
cinnamon essential oil
(*Cinnamomum verum*
or *Cinnamomum
zeylanicum*)

2 drops essential rose or
rose geranium oil

3.   Pour this hot oil and butter mixture into a mixing bowl, and mix with
a hand mixer or stand mixer for the best results. Slowly add the hot rose
water preparation to the oil while mixing on high. While mixing, add all the
essential oils until milky.

Store in a sterilized glass jar in the refrigerator and use within 2 weeks for
best results.

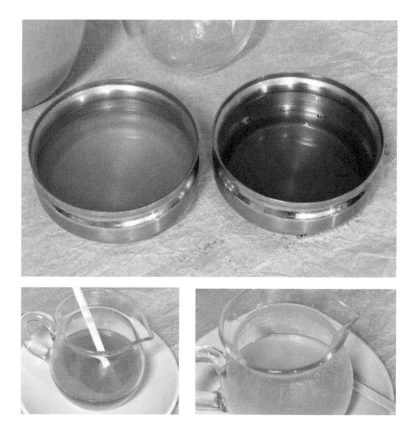

---

* Made with sunflower oil for
best results

Apothecary Cannabis Rose Cold Cream

This is a thick, moisturizing cold cream reminiscent of the rose cold creams of the 1950s. This cold cream should remain refrigerated; cold processing makes the cold cream extremely refreshing when applied to the skin after a hot shower or spa. This cold cream is my favorite daily treat whenever I have a fresh batch on hand.

1. Combine rose water, lemon juice, and the aloe vera gel in the blender until smooth. Pour into a pan and heat to 175 degrees Fahrenheit (80 degrees Celsius).
2. Melt the kokum butter, mango seed butter, sunflower lecithin, and cannabis oil in a separate pan on the stove. Heat this mixture to 175 degrees Fahrenheit (80 degrees Celsius).
3. Pour this hot oil and butter mixture into a mixing bowl and mix with a hand mixer or stand mixer for the best results. Slowly add the hot rose water preparation to the oil while mixing on high. Add all the essential oils while mixing until the preparation is fully emulsified and creamy.
4. Refrigerate and allow to completely cool, typically 1 hour—the cream will stiffen up as it cools. After the cooling period, take the cream out of the refrigerator and whip it up again with a hand or stand mixer until it's very fluffy and creamy.
5. Store in a sterilized glass container in the refrigerator and use within 2 weeks for best results.

½ cup (120 milliliters) distilled rose water
½ teaspoon (2 milliliters) lemon juice
3 tablespoons (45 milliliters) aloe vera gel, scraped from the fresh leaf
1 tablespoon (15 milliliters) kokum butter
⅓ cup (78 milliliters) mango seed butter
1 teaspoon (5 grams) sunflower lecithin
¼ cup (60 milliliters) **Cannabis Foundation Oil*** (page 36)
1 drop True Ceylon cinnamon essential oil (*Cinnamomum verum* or *Cinnamomum zeylanicum*)
5 drops essential rose or rose geranium oil

* Made with sunflower oil for best results

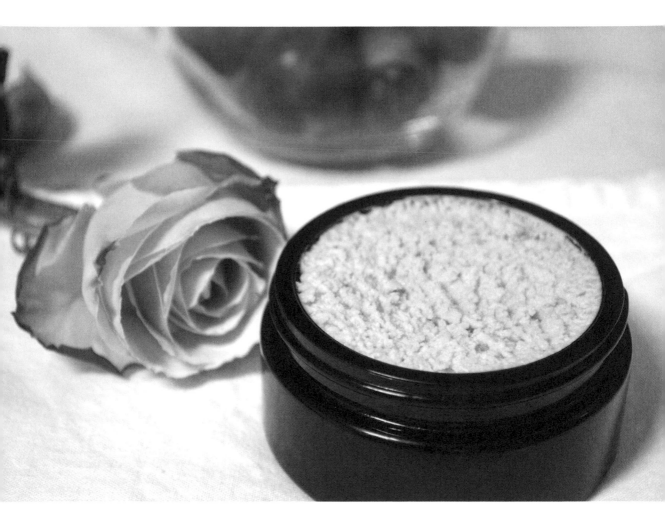

Recovery Pain Cream

This is a thick, medicated cream that's even better when used with a moist hot towel wrap.

This cream contains three intensive anti-inflammatory herbs: ginger, turmeric, and cannabis. It's really great for sports injuries and sore muscles. I love the healing warmth of this cream after a workout or exercise session. This recovery cream will add a temporary golden glow to the skin due to the presence of turmeric.

¼ cup (60 milliliters) orange flower water
½ teaspoon (2 milliliters) lemon juice
1 tablespoon (5 grams) turmeric powder
¼ cup (60 milliliters) aloe vera gel, scraped from the leaf
¼ cup (60 milliliters) kokum butter
1 teaspoon (5 grams) sunflower lecithin
½ cup (120 milliliters) **Cannabis Foundation Oil** (page 36)
10 drops essential ginger oil
1 drop any cinnamon oil
5 drops tulsi essential oil

1. In a blender, combine orange flower water, lemon juice, turmeric powder, and the aloe vera gel for a few seconds until thoroughly smooth. Pour into a pan on the stove and heat to 175 degrees Fahrenheit (80 degrees Celsius).
2. Melt the kokum butter, sunflower lecithin, and cannabis oil in a separate pan on the stove. Heat this mixture to 175 degrees Fahrenheit (80 degrees Celsius).
3. Pour hot oil and butter mixture into a mixing bowl and mix with a hand mixer or stand mixer for the best results. Slowly add the hot orange flower water and aloe vera preparation to the oil while mixing on high. Add all of the essential oils while mixing until creamy and smooth.

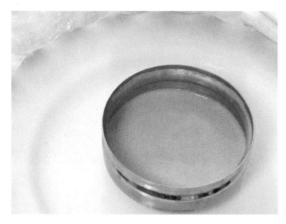

4. Refrigerate for 1 hour, then whip again on high for an extra-fluffy cream. This cream will stiffen as it cools in the refrigerator. Store this cream in the refrigerator and use within 2 weeks for best results.

First stage of cream emulsification

Thai Stick Lemongrass Lotion

3 stalks fresh lemongrass with the green cut away

½ cup (120 milliliters) aloe vera gel, scraped from the leaf

½ cup (120 milliliters) distilled water or spring water

½ teaspoon (2 milliliters) lemon juice

1 teaspoon (5 grams) sunflower lecithin

¼ cup (60 milliliters) mango seed butter

¼ cup (60 milliliters) **Cannabis Foundation Oil** (page 36)

Reminiscent of the earlier years of the drug war when the legendary Thai strains or "Thai Sticks" were a hot commodity, if you could get them! This lotion was named for a great sativa strain, so I use the **Cannabis Foundation Oil** from chapter 1, made with dried and ground Thai strains of cannabis flowers. This recipe uses both fresh lemongrass stalks and fresh aloe vera leaves. This lotion is not only a great moisturizer, but also a great bug repellent. And it's gentle on your skin!

1. Cut up the lemongrass stalks and scrape the gel from fresh aloe vera leaves. Blend the water and lemongrass stalks in a blender until almost smooth. Filter all of the solids from the liquid. Put the liquid back in the blender with the aloe vera gel and lemon juice and blend until smooth. Heat this liquid to 175 degrees Fahrenheit (80 degrees Celsius).

2. Melt sunflower lecithin, mango seed butter, and cannabis oil in a separate pan. Heat this mixture to 175 degrees Fahrenheit (80 degrees Celsius).

3. Pour this hot oil and butter mixture into a mixing bowl, and mix with a hand mixer or stand mixer for the best results. Slowly add the hot aloe vera, lemon juice, and lemongrass preparation to the oil while mixing on high until creamy and smooth.

4. Store this lotion in the refrigerator and use within 2 weeks for best results.

Kaneh Bosem Desert Caravan Cold Cream

This is a cooling recipe that incorporates some cinnamon from the **Kaneh Bosem Healing Oil** recipe. It's a great cold cream for hot and dry conditions.

1. In the blender, combine the lemon juice, orange flower water, and aloe vera until smooth. Heat this mixture in a pan on the stove to 175 degrees Fahrenheit (80 degrees Celsius).
2. Melt the sunflower lecithin, butter, and cannabis oil in a pan on the stove at 175 degrees Fahrenheit (80 degrees Celsius).
3. Pour this hot oil and butter mixture into a mixing bowl, and mix with a hand mixer or stand mixer for the best results. Slowly add the hot aloe vera and orange flower water preparation to the oil while mixing on high. Add all the essential oils while mixing until creamy and smooth.
4. Store this lotion in the refrigerator and use within 2 weeks.

½ teaspoon (2 milliliters) lemon juice
½ cup (120 milliliters) distilled orange flower water
¼ cup (60 milliliters) aloe vera gel, scraped from the leaf
1 teaspoon (5 grams) sunflower lecithin
½ cup (120 milliliters) mango seed butter
½ cup (120 milliliters) **Kaneh Bosem Healing Oil** (page 40)
3 drops bergaterpene-free orange or citron essential oil
2 drops carnation flower essential oil
5 drops henna flower essential oil

Simple (But Powerful) Cannabis Lotion

½ cup (120 milliliters)
Cannabis Foundation Oil* (page 36)
1 teaspoon (5 grams) sunflower lecithin
¼ cup (60 milliliters) preservative-free aloe vera juice
½ teaspoon (2 milliliters) lemon juice
any essential oils you prefer

A very simple-to-make cannabis lotion is created using the concentrated **Cannabis Foundation Oil** from chapter 1, along with just three other ingredients. Try it!

1. Gently heat the cannabis oil to 175 degrees Fahrenheit (80 degrees Celsius) then melt the sunflower lecithin in the oil preparation until dissolved. At the same time, warm the aloe vera juice and lemon juice to the same temperature as the oil preparation, 175 degrees Fahrenheit (80 degrees Celsius).

2. Pour the heated oil in a bowl and begin mixing with a whisk or hand mixer while slowly pouring in the heated aloe vera juice. Mix in the essential oils. You can see a milky lotion forming as the mixture begins its cooling process. Mix until fully emulsified and milky. Refrigerate immediately and allow to completely cool, typically about 1 hour.

3. After the refrigerated cooling period, take the lotion out and whip it up with a hand or stand mixer until extra creamy and smooth. Store in a sterilized glass jar in the refrigerator for up to 2 weeks.

TIP: Always discard any water-based spa preparation that begins to smell "off" or otherwise changes appearance or color, or if a preparation has been left out of the refrigerator for more than a few hours.

---

* The olive oil recipe from chapter 1 works best. You may also experiment using Herbal Spa Oil Jar aged oils or another cannabis oil herbal infusion.

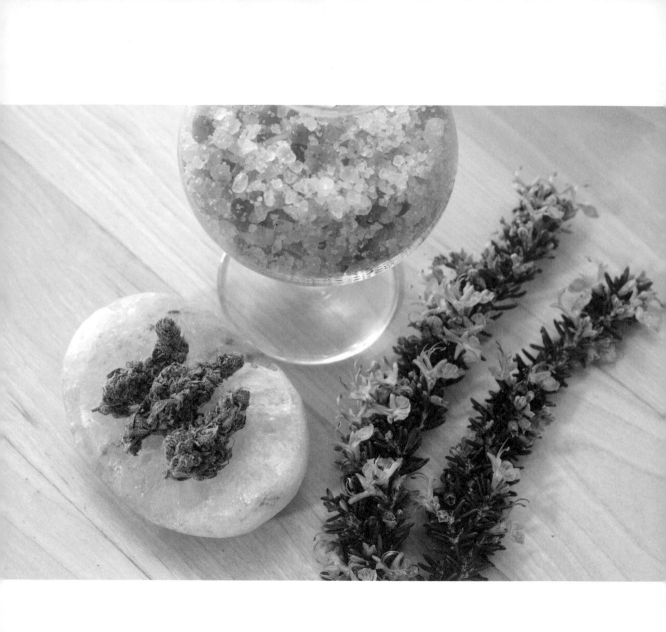

CHAPTER THREE:
LET'S GET HIGH
ON BATH SALTS

———————— 🍁 ————————

(No, really!)

There. I knew that would get your attention! But, I'm not talking about *those* bath salts. Cannabis won't turn you into a zombie, I promise!

These cannabis bath salts are soothing, anti-inflammatory, non-drying, and luscious on the skin. And if you're seeking pain relief from a number of conditions like arthritis, chronic headaches, cramps, or nerve pain, these baths will leave you refreshed and feeling fantastic.

It's hard to smile when you are in pain, but a smile is always guaranteed with every one of these baths.

Caveat: These bath preparations do have the potential to relax your muscles and induce euphoria depending on the concentration of cannabinoids used and the length of time you spend in the bath. Please avoid driving or operating heavy machinery after bathing. Allow 3 to 8 hours; the actual duration depends on the concentration of cannabinoids you've absorbed. These baths may also be adjusted so they have no psychoactive effect at all, while still providing benefits similar to topical lotions.

You can prepare the bath salts in any cannabinoid concentration you prefer; there is no upward limit. However, you may need to adjust other ingredients to ensure the cannabis oils have been fully emulsified. More than the suggested amount of cannabis can be wasteful. The effects of these baths have more to do with soaking time (exposure) than deploying super-concentrations of cannabinoids. That being said, if you are seeking maximum pain relieving benefits that include some euphoria, this bath formulation does require more cannabis than other spa preparations and even edibles.

You should spend as much time soaking in this bath as you feel is necessary. Based on the experiences of those who have tried these baths, the consensus is that you will begin to feel the benefits in 15 minutes, with typical soak times averaging between 30 and 60 minutes for maximum benefits. Wait at least 60 minutes after you have taken a bath to evaluate your level of sobriety.

The Bath Salts Story

I'm frequently asked how I came up with these bath salt recipes! Like a lot of other interesting inventions, it was somewhat by accident.

I've used many bath salts from the legal dispensaries, and I've attempted to make my own using standard bath bomb and salt techniques. The problem with these methods is that the cannabis oils either float on top of the water, for a not-so-lovely "ring around the tub," or they end up encapsulated in some form of starch. Neither results in a fully emulsified bath that really penetrates into your tissues.

I had previous knowledge of saponins as a potent surfactant that emulsifies oils and keeps them emulsified. Saponins also increase absorption of essential oils transdermally. With that in mind, I experimented with traditional folk herbal saponins like soapberries. I was very excited to experience the result after finishing my first soapberry cannabis bath base mixed with Himalayan pink salt.

I was initially aiming for the same kind of non-psychoactive pain relief I received from the lotion recipes. I soaked in the tub for about 1 hour before I was scheduled to drive to an appointment. Well, that was a wash, literally! About 15 minutes after getting out of that powerful bath, I was too euphoric to drive!

Now I'm more careful, of course!

The Key Features of the Bath Salts Recipe:

1.   **Emulsion and even distribution of oil in the formula.**
Emulsion is the process of combining oil and water by using a saponin and other ingredients—in this case, a surfactant providing saponins (*Sapindus mukorossi*), plus *mucilage* (aloe vera), and sunflower lecithin—to firm up the emulsion. The resulting oils stay emulsified and active when added to bathwater—no ring around the tub or wasted oils that float on the surface!

2.   **Fully decarboxylated cannabis oils and extracts.**
Decarboxylation is a chemical reaction that sheds carbon atoms from carbon chains when cannabinoids are heated to approximately 300 degrees Fahrenheit (150 degrees Celsius) for 30 minutes or more. All the bath recipes include this important step to ensure that the cannabinoids are fully bioactive.

3.   **A low-foaming formula that works well with salt crystals.**
These baths can be used in jetted tubs or soaking tubs. They are high in saponins derived from the soapberries and will not foam heavily in a jetted tub—you may see some light foaming, but it will dissipate fairly quickly.

Making cannabis bath salts is a two step process:
1.   Making the concentrated cannabis bath base.
2.   Adding the concentrated cannabis bath base to a salt and aloe vera mixture, then finishing by adding your selected essential oils and/or teas.

Making the Cannabis Bath Base

I start with fresh, authentic, dried, de-seeded *Sapindus mukorossi* berries. In chapter 1, I outlined what these berries are and where you can obtain them. They are part of the traditional Ayurvedic pharmacopoeia and have been used for thousands of years for skin and hair health. They're also noted for their anti-inflammatory and antimicrobial properties, which nicely complements the cannabis herb.

Soapberries are unique in the way that their saponins interact with cannabinoids in water, promptly emulsifying and evenly distributing them. This makes soapberries perfect for bath formulations that include cannabis. *Sapindus mukorossi* has the most important qualities necessary to create superior bath formulas for our purposes: it's low-foaming and high in saponins.

Do not substitute other surfactants or soap products.

Do not use any pre-prepared soapberry product.

Use only the raw product, and for best results, prepare the soapberries exactly according to this recipe.

Sapindus mukorossi has a distinctive, pleasant "cooked pineapple" or "apple cider vinegar" fragrance when it's cooked by itself. You may be able to detect the fragrance of cannabis before the scent of soapberries in a bath if you are not using additional herbs, such as citrus or lavender.

In the basic recipes, I prepare the bath base with citrus peels and lavender to round out the fragrance of the soapberries and cannabis. This enhances the aromatherapy experience of the custom bath recipes that follow. Bath bases prepared this way can also be used alone, with no additional essential oils or spices, for a virtually fragrance-free bath. You may also elect to omit citrus and lavender altogether; they are not required in the basic process that combines the bath base with bath salts to produce a fully-emulsified cannabis bath.

My bath recipes include mostly easy-to-source ingredients, detailed in chapter 1. I do include some exotic ingredients, like flower attars, which may be sourced from the resource guide at the end of this book (and online). The resource guide lists the sources I trust for authentic and fresh

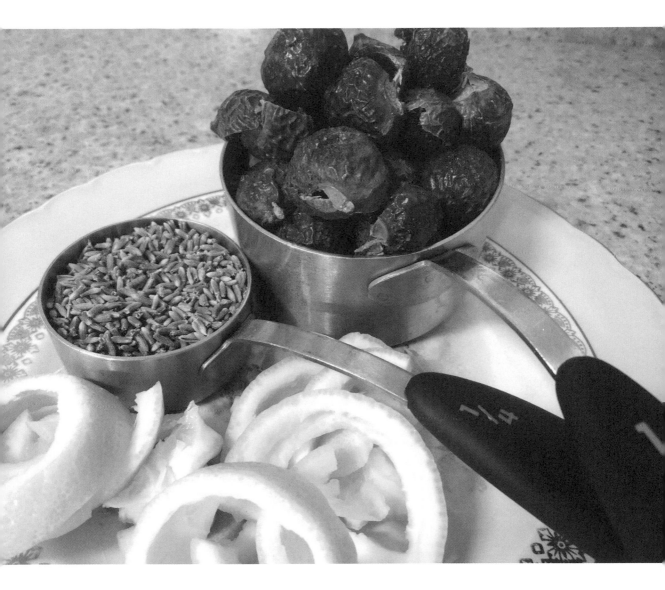

ingredients. These ingredients have worked well in my test kitchen when making each of the recipes.

This bath base is not shelf-stable and requires refrigeration. Failure to refrigerate can result in microbial contamination. This is a small-batch recipe that will make 3 to 5 baths, depending on your preference. This bath base can be frozen for up to 6 months.

These bath salts are a perishable product. While salt inhibits the growth of many bad organisms, it doesn't inhibit them all. To avoid microbial contamination, any bath salts you make should be refrigerated and used within 1 to 2 weeks for the best results.

My standard routine is to make five bath portions at a time. Each portion contains the cannabinoid equivalent of 1 gram of hashish, roughly the same as 3 grams of flower or 7 grams of trim. The suggested amounts in this recipe can vary depending on your preference; these bath recipes can be as intensive or as gentle as you like.

I enjoy immersing my entire body, head and all! The soapberry formulation makes these baths a great cleanser for hair and body. Rinse in the shower briefly after taking a bath, if you prefer.

½ teaspoon (2 grams) sunflower lecithin

½ –1 tablespoon (7–15 milliliters) olive or sunflower oil**

3–14 grams or more of potent, dried, and finely ground cannabis flowers *OR* 2–8 or more grams of hashish or keif *OR* 10–28 grams or more cannabis trim, ground

60 whole, de-seeded *Sapindus Mukorossi* berries (soapberry, aritha) split in half*

1 tablespoon (3 grams) dried lavender flowers *OR* a few fresh sprigs of fresh lavender flowers

citrus peels from 1 citrus fruit

1 quart (1 liter) water

2 tablespoons (30 milliliters) aloe vera gel, scraped from the leaf

---

* If you are creating a bath base that is at the higher end of cannabinoid concentration, use more soapberries for better emulsification. You may continue to add soapberries during the cooking process.

** The amount should be just enough to saturate the plant material or dissolve the concentrate material.

The Basic Cannabis Bath Base Recipe

Uses Dried and Finely Ground Cannabis Trim, Flowers, Hashish, or Keif

Splitting this bath base into five portions has the relieving and non-psychoactive effect of most cannabis lotions. Six or more portions is ideal if you have a low tolerance or have not used cannabis before and want smaller concentrations of cannabinoids. Three or fewer portions will intensify effects and may be psychoactive. Please plan your activities accordingly. Longer soak times will intensify the effects of any portion size you choose.

Makes 3 or more bath base portions

1. Melt the sunflower lecithin in the oil. Pour this hot oil over the cannabis and allow it to marinate while you prepare the soapberries.

2. Rinse the dried soapberries in warm water once quickly and drain. Add the soapberries, citrus peels, and lavender to a bowl.

3. Bring the water to a boil on the stove and add to the ingredients in the bowl. Allow this to sit on the counter, covered, overnight or 6–8 hours to extract the saponins and other essential ingredients from the herbs.

4. After this extraction, put the soapberry mixture on the stove and add the marinated cannabis and aloe vera gel that has been scraped from the fresh leaf. Cook this mixture at a low simmer and on medium heat while frequently mashing down and stirring until it reduces to about half as much liquid or less. This will take about 45–60 minutes. The plant material should be mushy and pulpy at the end of this process.

5. Remove and allow this to cool to a warm-to-the-touch temperature. Using a strainer or cloth bag, extract as much juice as possible from the mixture in a bowl. This is your first and strongest bath base mixture.

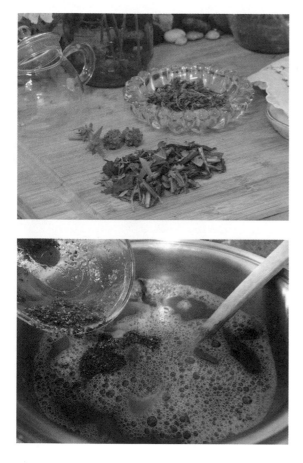
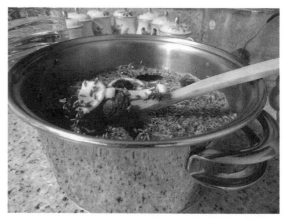

You should have about 1–2 cups (240–480 milliliters) of thick, gravy-like liquid. The soapberries and cannabis flower material left over will be set aside for a second extraction used in the poultice, wrap, foot, and hand soak recipes.

Additionally, you may use the second or even third extractions for a full bath. Extract again using 1 quart (1 liter) of boiling water, cool, and strain as before. Use this as a base for any of the bath recipes.

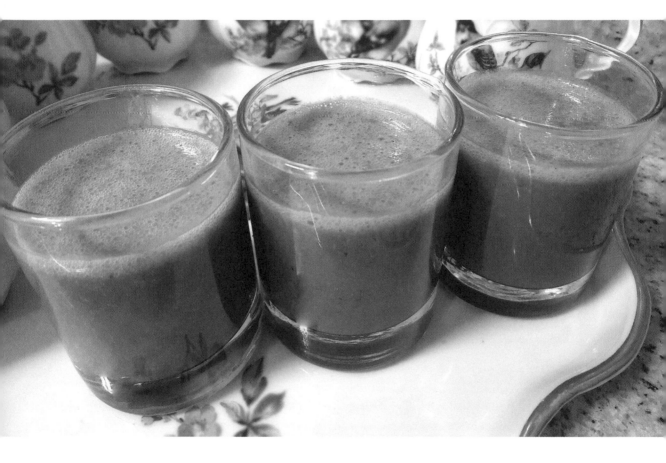

The Basic Cannabis Bath Base Recipe

Uses Full-Extract Decarboxylated Cannabis Oil ("Simpson Oil")

Full-extract cannabis oil is a fully decarboxylated cannabis oil that normally uses alcohol in the extraction process that is then boiled off to create a thick and concentrated tar-like oil. I explain more about the origins and popularity of this oil in chapter 1.

If you live in a location with legal cannabis dispensaries, there is a good chance you will be able to purchase this oil or have a caregiver make it for you.

This recipe is different than the basic bath base with raw cannabis because we do not need to take the oil through the long simmering process. The oil is thinned with olive or sunflower oil and lecithin and added right before the soapberries have boiled down to a thick liquid.

Splitting this bath base into five portions or more if you have a low tolerance or have not used cannabis before—thereby using smaller concentrations of cannabinoids—has the relieving and non-psychoactive effect of most cannabis lotions. Three or fewer portions will intensify effects and may be psychoactive. Please plan your activities accordingly. Longer soak times intensify the effects of any portion size you choose.

1. Melt the sunflower lecithin in the oil. Prepare the full-extract cannabis oil by melting it in the olive or sunflower oil and lecithin on low heat. Cover and set aside.
2. Rinse the dried soapberries in warm water once, quickly. Add the soapberries, citrus peels, and lavender to a bowl.
3. Bring the water to a boil and add to the ingredients in the bowl. Allow this to sit on the counter overnight or 6–8 hours to fully extract the saponins and other essential ingredients from the herbs.
4. After this extraction, put the soapberry mixture on the stove and cook on a low simmer while frequently mashing down and stirring until it becomes very pulpy and reduces to about ⅔ as much liquid or less. This will take about 30 minutes.

½ teaspoon (2 grams) sunflower lecithin

3–7 grams or more full-extract cannabis oil ("Simpson Oil")

½–1 tablespoon (7–15 milliliters) olive or sunflower oil, or a little more if necessary**

60 whole, de-seeded *Sapindus Mukorossi* berries (soapberry, aritha) split in half*

citrus peels from 1 citrus fruit

1 tablespoon (3 grams) dried lavender flowers *OR* a few fresh sprigs of fresh lavender flowers

1 quart (1 liter) water

2 tablespoons (30 milliliters) aloe vera gel, scraped from the leaf

------

* If you are creating a bath base that is at the higher end of cannabinoid concentration, use more soapberries for better emulsification.

** The addition of this oil should be just enough to dilute the full-extract cannabis oil well enough to make it a bit thinner.

5. Add the aloe vera gel that has been scraped from the leaf and the cannabis oil to the mixture on the stove, mash, and cook for about 15 minutes on low heat, until the oil emulsifies into the thick liquid. Remove and allow this to cool to a warm-to-the-touch temperature.

6. Using a strainer or cloth bag, extract as much juice as possible from the mixture in a bowl. This is your first and strongest bath base mixture.

You should have about 1 to 2 cups (240–480 milliliters) of thick liquid. As with the raw cannabis bath base, the leftover pulp can be used again in soaks, poultices, and even in another extraction for a full bath.

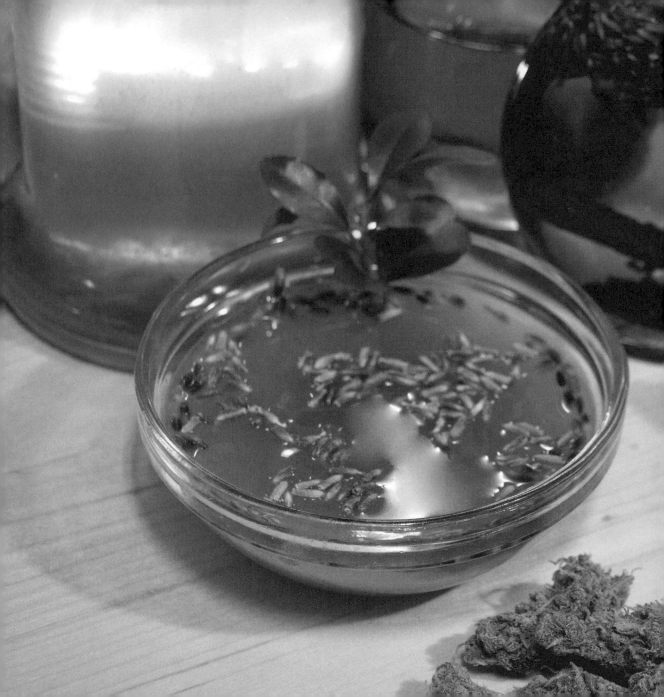

The Bath Salt and Tea Recipes

You will be adding essential oils and herbs at this point. The bath base is ideal to work with when it's still slightly warm. If you have previously frozen bath base portions, warm them up before making the bath salt recipes.

The Basic Bath Salt Recipe

The bath salt recipes that follow are all variations on this basic recipe.

Makes one bath

1. Using a large mortar and pestle or large glass mixing bowl, pour in all of the salt.
2. Scrape the gel from the aloe leaf and mash the aloe vera gel into the salt until dissolved.

1–2 cups (250–500 grams) coarse Himalayan pink salt, ancient salt, or sea salt for large soaking or jetted tubs
OR ½ cup–1 cup (125–250 grams) coarse Himalayan pink salt, ancient salt, or sea salt, for average-sized tubs
2 tablespoons (30 milliliters) aloe vera gel, scraped from the leaf
1 portion **Cannabis Bath Base** (page 84)
assorted essential oils, if desired

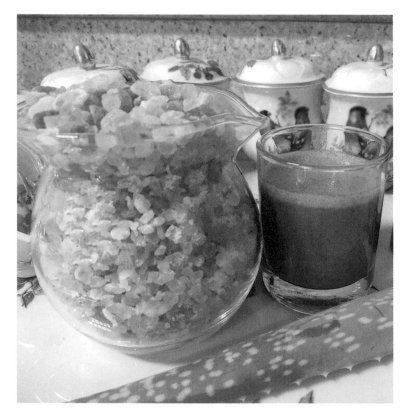

3. Add 1 portion of the cannabis bath base.

4. Add drops of the essential oils of your choice and gently fold into the mixture.

That's it! Refrigerate for up to 2 weeks, freeze for up to 6 months, or use immediately. I enjoy using spices or herbal teas in the recipes that follow. Brew these in a separate pan and add to the mixture after boiling with medium heat and reducing the liquid to about ¼ cup (60 milliliters).

It's also important to note that the final result in your tub will have a different fragrance than the final concentrated bath salt portion. The scents of the soapberry, lemon peels, and lavender dissipate to reveal the fragrance of the other ingredients. And again, if your preference is a virtually fragrance-free bath, make this basic bath salt recipe with no additional essential oils, herbal teas, or spices.

TIP: To preserve the integrity of the essential oils in these bath recipes, you'll need to use the baths immediately or put these baths in bottles or jars and refrigerate as soon as possible. Keep them tightly sealed.

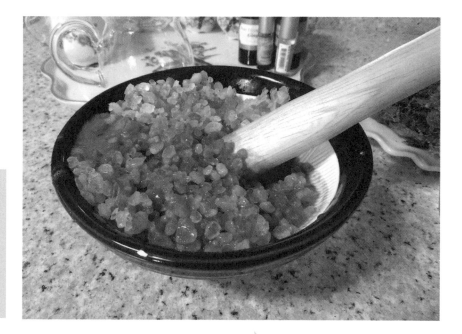

The Moonshine Bath

My grandmother used to make a cake called Moonshine Cake. It didn't actually have any alcohol in it, but it hails from the era of 1920s prohibition. It's a decadent and delicately scented white cake. She passed down her tattered recipe card to me many years ago, and that's the inspiration for this bath recipe. It's totally decadent, just like the cake. Celebrate the end of cannabis prohibition today with this Moonshine Bath!

This recipe uses the rare essential oils jasmine and carnation. These are among the most luxurious essential oils available and give this bath a distinctive floral note using just a few drops.

In the original version of this recipe, and some of the other recipes in this book, I used an amber paste that I loved; however, this ingredient proved to be too difficult to source consistently. This recipe now contains carnation flower essential oil, which imparts the spicy and resinous floral notes that lift this bath even higher!

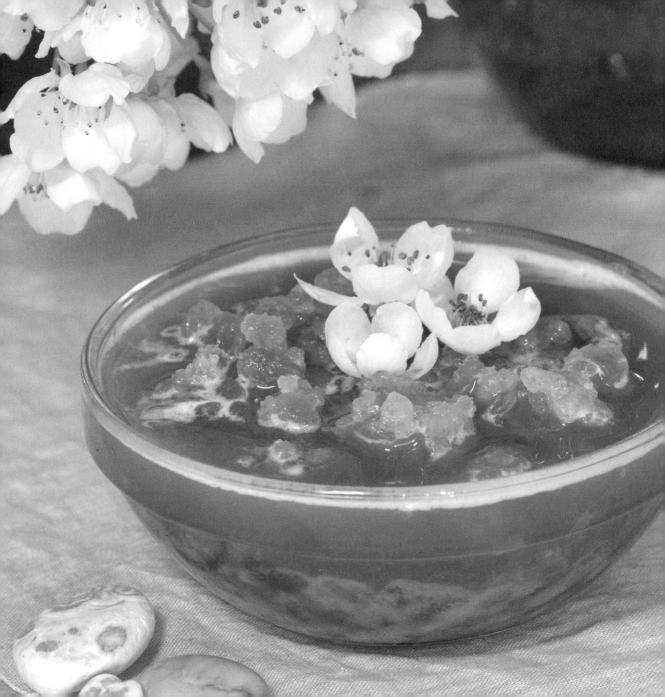

Makes one bath

1. Using a large mortar and pestle or large glass mixing bowl, pour in all of the salt. Scrape the gel from the aloe leaf and mash the aloe vera gel into the salt until dissolved.

2. In a pan on the stove, add the ginger, white tea, scraped vanilla bean, water, and boil using medium heat until there is only about ¼ cup (60 milliliter) of concentrated liquid. Cool and strain.

3. Add the bath base portion and the cooled spice and tea liquid to the salt while stirring.

4. Add the essential oils and vanilla seed pulp as the last step and fold in gently.

Your finished bath salt should be wet to semi-liquid. Use immediately or store in the refrigerator. Seal this in a tight container in the refrigerator for up to 2 weeks or in the freezer for up to 6 months.

1–2 cups (250–500 grams) coarse Himalayan pink salt, ancient salt, or sea salt for large soaking or jetted tubs
OR ½ cup–1 cup (125–250 grams) coarse Himalayan pink salt, ancient salt, or sea salt, for average-sized tubs
2 tablespoons (30 milliliters) aloe vera gel, scraped from the leaf
1 thumb fresh ginger, chopped
1 bag (2 grams) white tea
1 vanilla bean, scraped of seeds*
2 cups (480 milliliters) water
1 portion **Cannabis Bath Base** (page 84)
2 drops jasmine essential oil
2 drops carnation essential oil
2 drops frankincense essential oil

---

* Set aside the seed pulp and scraped bean separately.

The Recovery Bath

1–2 cups (250–500 grams) coarse Himalayan pink salt, ancient salt, or sea salt for large soaking or jetted tubs
OR ½ cup–1 cup (125–250 grams) coarse Himalayan pink salt, ancient salt, or sea salt, for average-sized tubs

2 tablespoons (30 milliliters) aloe vera gel, scraped from the leaf

¼ cup (60 grams) fresh grated turmeric root *OR* 1 tablespoon (5 grams) turmeric powder

1 cup (240 milliliters) water

1 portion **Cannabis Bath Base** (page 84)

5 drops ginger essential oil

2 drops lavender essential oil

5 drops rosemary essential oil

2 drops peppermint oil

1 drop palo santo essential oil

This bath is not for the faint of heart. This is a bath salt that I have personally employed against the evil pain of autoimmune disease; this bath is also great for all kinds of recovery situations, including sports injury recovery. I've reformulated this recipe to include palo santo essential oil. Palo santo is renowned for its purifying and healing attributes, but should only be used in small amounts due to its powerful fragrance.

This bath also contains raw turmeric root in quantities that may stain your skin a very slight golden color. If you have a tan or darker skin, this bath will make you glow! But if you have lighter skin, you may notice a slight golden color. It doesn't last long, but it will be present.

Turmeric is an essential part of this bath because of its anti-inflammatory properties. You may omit this ingredient, but the results may vary.

Makes one bath

1. Using a large mortar and pestle or large glass mixing bowl, pour in all of the salt. Scrape the gel from the aloe leaf and mash the aloe vera gel into the salt until dissolved.

2. In a pan on the stove, add the turmeric and water and boil until there is about ¼ cup (60 milliliters) of concentrated liquid. Allow this to cool and strain if necessary.

3. Add the cannabis bath base and turmeric tea to the salt while stirring.

4. Add the essential oils as the last step and fold in gently.

Your finished bath salt should be wet to semi-liquid. Use immediately or store in the refrigerator. Seal in an airtight container in the refrigerator for up to 2 weeks or in the freezer for up to 6 months.

Sultana's Bath

Inspired by the hammam traditions of the Middle East and Sufi poetry, Sultana's Bath is the perfect romance and relaxation bath.

This bath uses rose essential oil, known as "attar of rose," henna flower attar, carnation flower essential oil, and spices for an intoxicating scent that is like an oasis of beauty and love. The earthy scent of the henna flower is included in this formula for warmth and grounding. Henna is renowned in the desert climates and is used there for perfumery, sunscreen, skin health, and beauty.

Makes one bath

1. Using a large mortar and pestle or large glass mixing bowl, pour in all of the salt. Scrape the gel from the aloe leaf and mash the aloe vera gel into the salt until dissolved.
2. In a pan on the stove, combine the spices, orange peels, and water. Boil using medium heat until there is only about ¼ cup (60 milliliters) of concentrated liquid. Cool and strain.
3. Add the cannabis bath base and spice liquid to the salt and stir.
4. Add the essential oils as the last step and fold in gently.

Your finished bath salt should be wet to semi-liquid. Use immediately or store in the refrigerator. Seal in a tight container in the refrigerator for up to 2 weeks or in the freezer for up to 6 months.

1–2 cups (250–500 grams) coarse Himalayan pink salt, ancient salt, or sea salt for large soaking or jetted tubs
OR ½ cup–1 cup (125–250 grams) coarse Himalayan pink salt, ancient salt, or sea salt, for average-sized tubs
2 tablespoons (30 milliliters) aloe vera gel, scraped from the leaf
1 cinnamon stick
5 cardamom pods, broken
3 clove buds
10 threads saffron
dried blood orange peels from 1 orange or regular orange peels
2 cups (480 milliliters) water
1 portion **Cannabis Bath Base** (page 84)
2 drops rose or geranium rose essential oil
2 drops henna flower attar
1 drop carnation flower essential oil
2 drops frankincense essential oil
1 drop myrrh essential oil

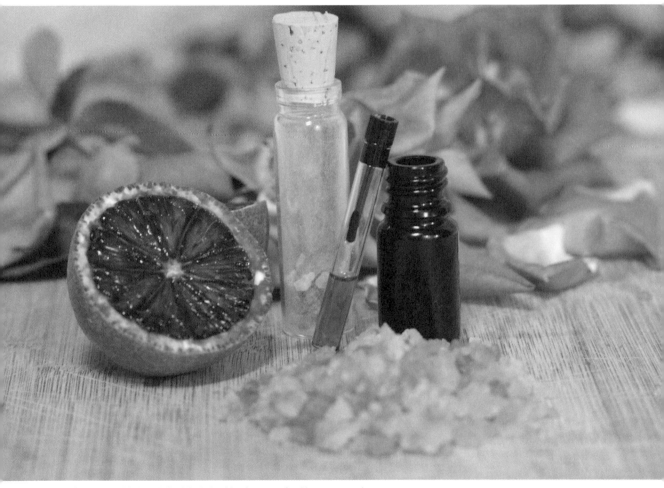

The exotic fragrance of Sultana's Bath includes blood orange, frankincense, myrrh, and henna flower attar.

Shiva's Bath

A spicy, citrusy, and slightly floral bath inspired by the Hindu deity who also loves the sacred cannabis herb. This bath has a strong lingam vibration for the warrior or the wounded. Perfect for man or woman, Shiva's Bath features the davana flower, which is offered to Shiva as garlands. Davana adds a spicy, fruity floral aroma said to smell slightly different on everyone! Davana flower essential oil possesses a bold fragrance, so less is more in most recipes that include a blend of essential oils.

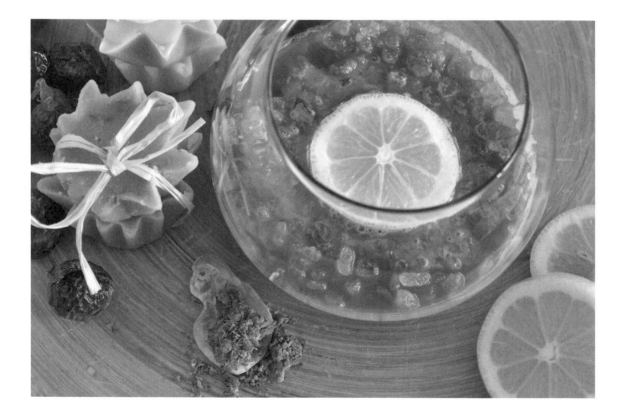

1–2 cups (250–500 grams) coarse Himalayan pink salt, ancient salt, or sea salt for large soaking or jetted tubs
OR ½ cup–1 cup (125–250 grams) coarse Himalayan pink salt, ancient salt, or sea salt, for average-sized tubs
2 tablespoons (30 milliliters) aloe vera gel, scraped from the leaf
2 cinnamon sticks
1 star anise
1 cardamom pod, cracked
1 thumb fresh ginger, chopped
OR 1 tablespoon ginger powder
1 cup dried blood orange peels or regular orange peels
1 portion **Cannabis Bath Base** (page 84)
2 drops jasmine essential oil
5 drops lemon essential oil
1 drop davana flower essential oil
1 drop patchouli essential oil
1 tablespoon (15 grams) or 2 bags black tea
2 cups (480 milliliters) water

Makes one bath

1. Using a large mortar and pestle or large glass mixing bowl, pour in all of the salt. Scrape the gel from the aloe leaf and mash the aloe vera gel into the salt until dissolved.
2. In a pan on the stove, add all of the spices, ginger, and orange peels to the water. Boil using medium heat until there is only about ¼ cup (60 milliliters) of concentrated liquid. Cool and strain.
3. Add the cannabis bath base and spice liquid to the salt and stir.
4. Add the essential oils as the last step and fold in gently.

Your finished bath salt should be wet to semi-liquid. Use immediately or store in the refrigerator. Seal this in a tight container in the refrigerator for up to 2 weeks or in the freezer for up to 6 months.

Cannabis Bath Tea

This recipe couldn't be more satisfying! The leftover pulp from making the **Cannabis Bath Base** can be used to make single-serving bath teas. I like to make three bath teas at once then use one right away and freeze the other two. You can get as creative as you like with this recipe and use both fresh and dried herbs, essential oils, fruits, and flowers in your bath tea bag.

Makes 3–5 bath teas

1. In a large bowl, combine everything thoroughly. Fill each of the muslin or hemp bags half full with a portion of the bath tea, leaving plenty of space for the herbs to expand and release their vital ingredients during the bath.
2. Use right away or store in a freezer container for up to 6 months.

This bath tea gives the best results if it is used in warm to hot baths. Always begin by preparing your bath tea with very, very hot water, swishing the bag around, and allow it to release into the hot water for 10 minutes or more before filling the rest of your tub with water, adjusting it to a temperature that is comfortable for you. Leave the tea bag in the water as you soak. You can use the bag to massage or scrub your skin during the bath!

leftover pulp from **Cannabis Bath Base** (page 84)

10–15 *Sapindus Mukorossi* soapberries, cracked into small pieces

½ cup (120 grams) chopped, fresh, whole aloe vera leaf

2 cups (500 grams) herbs, essential oils, fruits, and flowers of your choice*

drawstring muslin or hemp fabric tea or infusion bags

freezer storage container

* Chop and bruise everything, but do not liquefy.

Cannabis Soaks and Plunges

That bowl of leftover maceration from making cannabis bath base is now ready to be used to make these fabulous soaks!

After you extract most of the liquid from the plant material for your bath base portions, you'll want to do one more extraction to release all of the plant saponins, fragrances, and nutrients along with the remaining cannabinoids. This extraction is perfect for foot spas and soaks and for my signature hand plunge technique. You may also extract one portion from the leftover maceration for use in a full bath with salt. Additionally, in chapter 4 there are more recipes for poultices and wraps that use this second extraction of the bath base.

Cannabis Soak Base

This extraction makes 3 portions.

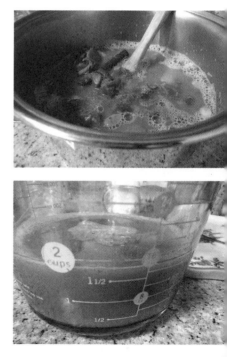

1. Add all leftover plant material, including any tea material, to a pot with 1 quart (1 liter) of boiling water.
2. Agitate and allow this to cool for 2–3 hours. Strain.
3. Split into 3 portions.

Refrigerate if not used immediately and use within 2 weeks or freeze for up to 6 months.

The Ultimate Foot Spa

This is for everyone who has spent one or more days on their feet. This foot bath recipe utilizes one portion of the second extraction of the leftover cannabis bath base maceration.

I include my special essential oil formula here for hot, tired, and painful feet, but you can add your own essential oils to make the perfect custom foot bath for you. I like this bath in a bubbly foot spa or just a basin; either way, it's an awesome foot soak that will have you walking on clouds.

Makes one foot bath

1. Add the gel from the aloe vera leaf and essential oils to the salt and thoroughly combine.
2. Add the salt to 1 portion of the bath base.
3. Prepare your foot spa or basin with any temperature of water you prefer. Add the foot soak mixture to the water.

Soak for any length of time! This recipe works well in jet foot spas as well as basin soakers.

2 tablespoons (30 milliliters) aloe vera gel, scraped from the leaf

3 drops ginger essential oil

2 drops peppermint essential oil

2 drops lemon essential oil

¼ cup (60 grams) coarse Himalayan pink salt, ancient salt, or sea salt

1 portion **Cannabis Soak Base** (page 99)

1 cup (240 milliliters) boiling water

1–2 quarts (1–2 liters) cold, warm, or hot water*

---

* Your foot bath can be any temperature that you like, including cool, but 1 cup of boiling water must be added first to aid the mixture in dissolving fully in the water.

The Ultimate Hand Plunge

2 tablespoons
(30 milliliters) aloe
vera gel, scraped from
the leaf
1 cup (240 milliliters)
boiling water + enough
water to fill the sink
and basin
3 drops ginger essential oil
1 drop palo santo essential
oil
2 drops frankincense
essential oil
1 portion **Cannabis Soak
Base** (page 99)

Arthritic hands begone! If you've ever lived with painful and stiff hands, or know someone who does, this hand bath gets right to the pain without any of the psychoactive effects that a full bath may have.

This bath uses a portion of the second extraction and should be made following the same steps as the foot bath. Prepare a deep sink or basin with water as hot as is comfortable for you. You'll want to soak your hands for 15 minutes or longer to get the most benefit from this hand plunge.

1. Add the gel from the aloe vera leaf to 1 cup (240 milliliters) of boiling water and stir.
2. Add the desired essential oils to the cannabis soak base.
3. Fill a sink or basin with water at your desired temperature. Add the aloe vera water and the cannabis soak base. Plunge your hands into the water and agitate to dissolve all salts. Continue to soak and massage your hands underwater for 15 minutes or longer.

TIP: I like to reheat the soak water throughout the day and use it multiple times before discarding on those days when my hands need more intensive care. Do this and your hands will thank you!

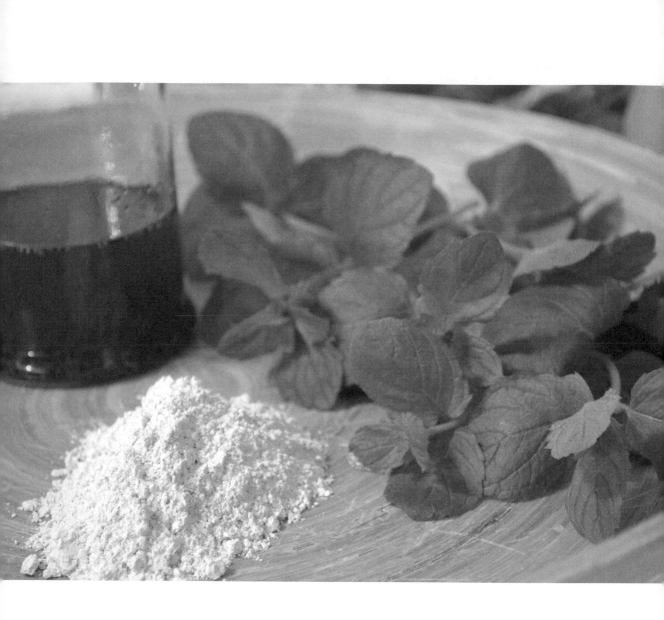

CHAPTER FOUR: LET'S GET WELL ON WRAPS, MASKS, AND POULTICES

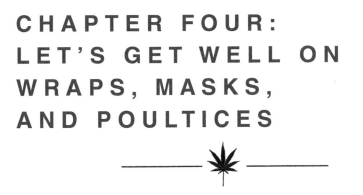

Cannabis works with wraps, masks, and poultices in ways that are similar to lotions and balms. The difference lies in their ability to be more spot-intensive, and you get the added benefits of detoxifying clay and additional healing herbs in these recipes.

Wraps and Poultices

"Poultice" typically consists of one or more of these techniques:

1. An application of herbal pastes, much like a mask
2. An application of herbal teas soaked in gauze or soft hemp fabric and wrapped around a limb or other body part
3. A mixture of oils and/or extracts that are applied to an area and covered with cloth bandages or herbs.

Poultices are one of my favorite ways to use cannabis as an herbal medicine. If you don't have time for a cannabis bath, a poultice can be the perfect substitute for the more intensive pain relief, especially for joint and muscle pain. Also poultices work great for burns and other skin injuries.

The Headache Poultice

My favorite way to medicate a nasty headache is with cannabis. There are so many ways to use cannabis this way, and a headache poultice ranks right up there—especially when the pain is the throbbing variety in the front of the head or when due to eye strain.

½ portion **Cannabis Bath Base** (page 84)
1 bunch fresh mint leaves
1 bowl ice chips
a washcloth or a washcloth-sized piece of absorbent fabric
½ cup (120 milliliters) cold water

1. Combine the cannabis bath base, mint leaves, and a few ice chips in a blender and blend until smooth. Strain the liquid through a cloth bag and add it to a bowl with a few ice chips to keep the liquid cool.
2. Dip the washcloth into the cold liquid, and gently squeeze just enough so it's not "drippy" but still retains much of the liquid. Fold and place over your eyes, forehead, or temples. This poultice should remain until it warms from your body heat, then dip it again in the cold liquid and repeat.

The unused poultice liquid can be frozen in an ice tray and used in single portions that are thawed out as needed.

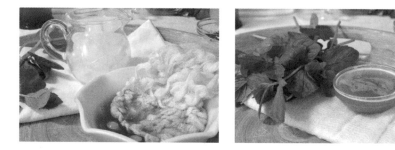

Herbal Tea Wrap

2 cups (480 milliliters)
  water
¼ cup (10 grams)
  chamomile flowers
  OR 10 bags chamomile
  tea
1 cinnamon stick
1 thumb ginger, chopped
¼ cup (60 milliliters) fresh
  aloe vera gel, scraped
  from the leaf
1 portion **Cannabis Bath
  Base** (page 84)
long pieces of clean and
  dry gauze, muslin, or
  soft hemp
several dry towels for
  wrapping

Don't have time for a cannabis bath, but need some really intensive relaxation and pain relief that's fast and also free of any psychoactive effects? Herbal tea poultice wraps really fit the bill!

This wrap uses one portion of the cannabis bath base described in chapter 3. You can make these cannabis bath base portions and freeze them for use in the bath and soak recipes, as well as the poultices.

1. With the water, brew the chamomile flowers, cinnamon, and ginger into a very strong tea and strain.
2. Add this hot liquid to the aloe vera and cannabis bath base in a blender, then transfer to a pan and gently heat until hot, but not hot enough to burn your fingers when dipping gauze or fabric into the liquid.
3. Dip the clean pieces of fabric into the liquid, then wrap them around sore muscles and joints.
4. Wrap a clean, preferably warm towel around the wet fabric and allow this to remain for at least 20 minutes.

Leftover liquid can be refrigerated for no more than 2 weeks. Reheat to the temperature of a cup of tea to repeat the wrap again.

Sunburn Poultice

This is the perfect cooling poultice that draws out heat and promotes healing of the skin. It uses the leftover cannabis plant material from making the concentrated cannabis oil in chapter 1.

leftover plant material from making the **Cannabis Foundation Oil** (page 36)

¼ cup (60 milliliters) fresh aloe vera gel, scraped from the leaf

1 stalk fresh lemongrass

¼ cup (60 milliliters) orange flower water

long pieces of clean and dry gauze, muslin, or soft hemp

1 cup (240 milliliters) very cold green tea

1. In a blender, combine the leftover cannabis plant material, aloe vera, lemongrass stalk, and orange flower water until smooth and frothy.
2. Apply this liquid plant paste to the affected areas. Dip the cloth strips in the cold green tea and loosely wrap the areas where the paste has been applied.
3. Leave on for 20 minutes or more, then remove the paste along with the cloth wrapping. Follow with a cool shower.

Unused paste can be frozen in an ice tray, and then used in single portions thawed out as needed.

Quick Wrap with Leftover Bath Base Herbs

2 cups (480 milliliters) boiling water
leftover pulp from making the **Cannabis Bath Base** (page 84)
a few drops of any essential oil
long pieces of clean and dry gauze, muslin, or soft hemp
several dry towels for wrapping

Got a pile of soapberries and herbs that haven't been extracted a second time yet? You can make a really great therapeutic cannabis wrap!

1. Add the boiling water to the leftover pulp. Allow this to stand for 30 minutes, then strain or squeeze through a cloth bag. Add essential oils to the liquid if desired.

2. You can use this liquid for a hot or cold wrap. Warm or cool the liquid for any application you choose.

3. Dip the gauze or other fabric into the liquid and apply to the affected area. You may wrap with a dry and hot towel for a deeper penetration of the healing benefits of this herbal liquid.

Leftover liquid can be refrigerated for no more than 2 weeks. Reheat to the temperature of a cup of tea to repeat the hot wrap or use straight from the refrigerator for a cooling wrap.

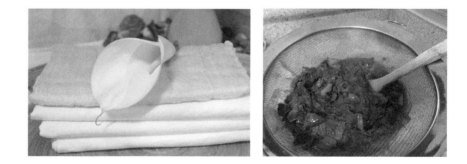

Herbal and Clay Masks

Apothecary Cannabis Rose Face and Body Mask

Based on the **Apothecary Cannabis Rose** series of lotions and balms, this face mask uses Ayurvedic herbs such as powdered rose petals and rose water to create a moisturizing—but not greasy—face mask that will minimize fine lines, making your skin as soft and smooth as rose petals.

1. Combine cannabis oil, aloe vera, lemon juice, and rose water in a blender. Slowly add the liquid to the powdered rose petals until the consistency is similar to mashed potatoes.

2. Apply to face, chest, arms, and legs and allow this to remain as long as you like; this mask is great for balancing and moisturizing normal to dry skin.

2 tablespoons (30 milliliters) **Cannabis Foundation Oil** (page 36)

¼ cup (60 milliliters) fresh aloe vera gel, scraped from the leaf

1 teaspoon (5 milliliters) lemon juice

½ cup (120 milliliters) rose water

½ cup (70 grams) powdered rose petals

Invigorating Cannabis Citrus Flower Mask

2 tablespoons
(30 milliliters)
**Cannabis Foundation
Oil** (page 36)
¼ cup (60 milliliters) fresh
aloe vera gel, scraped
from the leaf
1 teaspoon (5 milliliters)
lemon juice
½ cup (120 milliliters)
orange flower water
½ cup (70 grams)
powdered lemon rind

This refreshing mask is great for oily or normal skin. It also doubles as a refresher in hot weather for all skin types!

The special ingredient here, apart from cannabis, is powdered lemon rind, which has exfoliating and regenerating properties. Combined with cannabis, it is an invigorating and healing experience for your skin.

1. Combine cannabis oil, aloe vera, lemon juice, and orange flower water in a blender until smooth and frothy. Slowly add the liquid to the powdered lemon peels until the consistency is similar to mashed potatoes.
2. Apply to face, chest, arms, and legs (wherever you desire refreshed and renewed skin) for 10–15 minutes and wash off.

Detoxifying Cannabis Clay

This recipe can use any sterilized food-grade mineral clay powder. These are commonly available at health-food stores. This clay can be used for both internal and external purposes.

This recipe is a purifying treatment, perfect right before one of the cannabis baths from chapter 3. Apply the clay and allow to dry. Prepare the cannabis bath salts as shown in chapter 3 and add to very warm bath water.

¼ cup (60 milliliters) fresh aloe vera gel, scraped from the leaf
½ cup (120 milliliters) very concentrated green tea liquid
1 teaspoon (5 milliliters) lemon juice
2 tablespoons (30 milliliters) **Cannabis Foundation Oil** (page 36)
½ cup (70 grams) sterilized powdered mineral clay

1.   Combine the aloe vera, green tea, lemon juice, and cannabis oil in a blender until smooth and frothy.
2.   Slowly add to the powdered clay and mix until creamy.
3.   Store in a closed container in the refrigerator for up to three days.

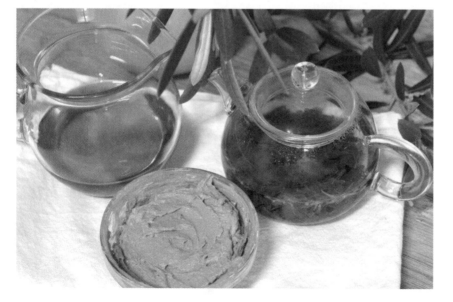

Pain Zap Clay

1 teaspoon (5 milliliters) lemon juice

¼ cup (60 milliliters) fresh aloe vera gel, scraped from the leaf

⅔ cup (158 milliliters) distilled or spring water

3 tablespoons (45 milliliters) **Cannabis Foundation Oil** (page 36)

½ cup (70 grams) sterilized powdered mineral clay

1 tablespoon (5 grams) turmeric powder

1 tablespoon (5 grams) ginger powder

pinch of powdered cloves

pinch of black pepper powder

pinch of powdered cinnamon

pinch of cayenne pepper

Inspired by the array of spices in my favorite Indo-Pakistani cuisine, which are so healing and anti-inflammatory, this pain-zapping clay is one of my favorites.

Do not use on your face or near any mucous membranes, as this clay contains spices and herbs that are warming on the skin but extremely hot if you get them in your eyes or mouth. Do not use on open wounds. If you do get the clay anywhere uncomfortable, rinse with regular milk.

This clay is great for aching backs, swollen joints, swollen feet, etc. It's the perfect pain-relieving treatment to use before taking the Recovery Bath from chapter 3. After the clay dries, immediately submerge your body in this warm bath—there's no need to wash the clay off ahead of time. This clay can also be used on feet or hands submerged in a full bath, the hand plunge bath, or with a foot spa from chapter 3.

1. Combine the lemon juice, aloe vera, water, and cannabis oil in a blender until smooth and frothy.
2. Combine the clay and all powdered spices thoroughly before slowly adding the liquid.
3. Use a hand or stand mixer to whip the mixture until fluffy.
4. Store in a closed container in the refrigerator for up to 3 days.

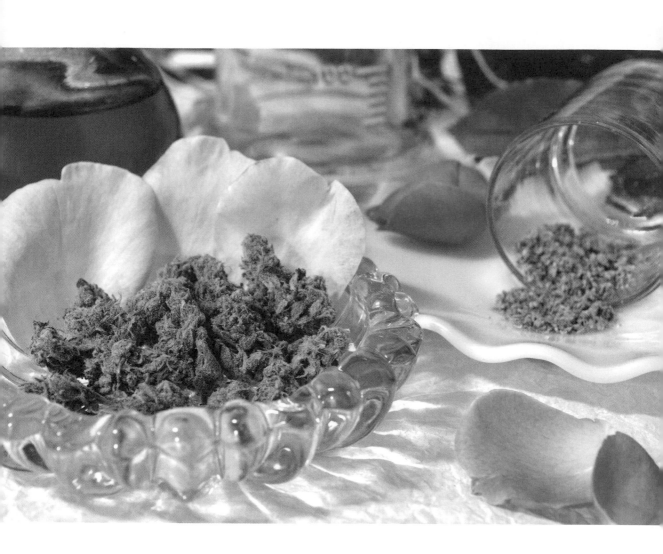

CHAPTER FIVE: AROMATHERAPY, TEA, BHANG, AND SMOOTHIES

Delicious things for your spa day or any day! Try these along with other treatments, like a bath or massage, for a truly luxurious cannabis spa experience.

Cannabis Aromatherapy

Living in a legal or medical cannabis state means that you have a lot to choose from! New strains are always being created by growers to express even more flavor in the end product. Cannabis naturally expresses many different flavors through terpene and flavonoid production in the plant itself. I've had cannabis that's tasted like lemons, chocolate, spices, oranges, grape soda, mangoes, and more.

Cannabis tasting can be as complex as tasting fine wines or cuisine. Enhancing your cannabis aromatherapy experience is what this chapter is all about. Smoking is out. It stinks, it's messy, and the charred particles are not good for your lungs. There are two really great ways to enjoy cannabis aromatherapy. Each one has its advantages:

A vaporizer—You've probably seen these. They come in box and forced-air models usually. They can also be in the form of a pen or other handheld device.

Vaporizers that handle ground flowers are fantastic when you really want to taste all the flavors the cannabis flower has to offer. Some vaporizers also handle cannabis essential oils and waxes.

A skillet or nail—Vapor bell skillets are relatively new devices that attach to a water pipe. They were originally created to serve "dabs" of essential cannabis oils and waxes.

But they do more than that. Skillets are also great for vaporizing finely ground cannabis flowers or keif. You can see how clean the residue actually is by the way your water pipe looks. When you smoke out of a water pipe, the residue left in the pipe is black, charred, and tar-like. When you use a skillet, the residue in your water pipe is clean like the residue from a vaporizer because skillets vaporize all of the essential oils quickly and cleanly, without any free radicals entering the pipe or your lungs.

Skillets also operate at a higher temperature than a vaporizer. Many people prefer the medicinal effects of cannabinoids that are smoked as opposed to vaped. Skillets produce a vapor that has the same efficiency as smoked cannabis due to these higher temperatures.

While skillets work beautifully with finely ground cannabis flowers and keif, they do not enhance the flavor experience the way vaporizers do. Cannabis flowers sauteed on a skillet have a more plain and neutral flavor. This is likely due to the very high temperature of the skillet plate.

Your glass bubbler or water pipe can host many different kinds of essential flavors and fragrances in the water to create a unique experience using a vapor bell skillet for cannabis aromatherapy.

What are cannabis essential oils and waxes and how are they used?

Cannabis essential oils and resins can be extracted using ethanol, petrochemical solvents such as butane, or natural solvents like carbon dioxide (CO_2), among others. Cannabis essential oils and resins are made using the same solvents—and in many cases, the same techniques—used by the mainstream aromatherapy industry.

As you can imagine, some solvents are not popular with many in the cannabis community, and they are also quite controversial in the mainstream aromatherapy community. I avoid essential oils and resins made with petrochemical solvents and recommend only eco-friendly and alcohol extraction processes.

Cannabis essential oils can be 70 percent or higher in THC. Taking a cue from the mainstream aromatherapy industry where CO_2 has become quite popular, many cannabis dispensaries now offer CO_2-extracted oils. The cannabis oils retain the lovely flavonoids and terpenes along with the medicinal cannabinoids. This eco-friendly and healthier form of extraction produces superior cannabis essential oils in every way.

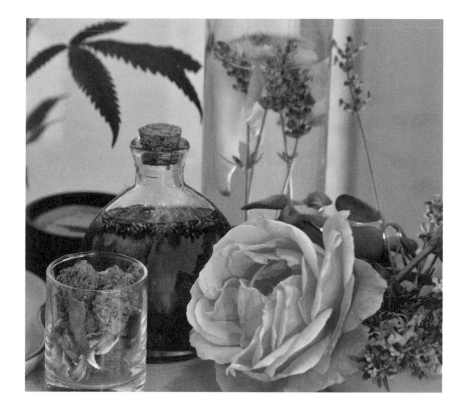

Potpourri and Essence Waters for Vape and Glass Service

Posh POTpourri

I like to call this technique Posh POTpourri—it's so easy and you can do it with spices you already have in your kitchen. And *wow*, does it raise the bar on cannabis flavor! You need just two weeks, dry whole spices, herbs, and a glass jar with a very tight lid. Some of the best Posh POTpourri I've ever had was stored with spices and herbs in miron glass for an entire month.

Posh POTpourri isn't just for storage flavor enhancement; it's something I regularly use on my own desk with the current selection of medicated herbs I'm using with my vaporizer.

Some of the dried spices and herbs that I've used for POTpourri blends are: vanilla beans, black peppercorns, cardamom pods, cinnamon sticks, citrus peels, roses, orange blossoms, cacao beans, coffee beans, ginger, and mint.

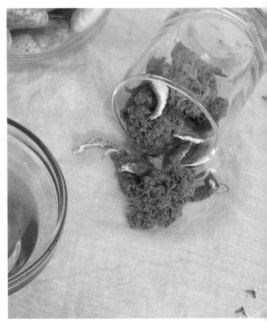

In my experience, what works best is to match the spices and herbs as closely as possible to the fragrance notes you discover in the cured cannabis flowers. For example, cookie, cake, and vanilla note strains are a favorite of mine to pair up with vanilla beans and even ginger. Citrus note strains hailing from Africa pair well with exotic citrus-like dried Buddha's Hand citron peel, dried rosebud, and black peppercorns. Be creative! Enhance the flavors and effects of the cannabis flower with any other spices and herbs that you love.

The Posh POTpourri is great to use if you have cannabis flowers that are good, but somewhat lacking in flavor—or they may need some refreshment if they've become too dry. Select the dried spices and herbs that are appealing to you and enjoy!

1. Prepare a clean glass jar by sterilizing and drying it thoroughly.
2. Fill the jar ⅓ full of the dried spice and herb blend of your choice.

It's important to note that you do not want to introduce moisture into this jar with your cannabis flowers. Your dried spice blend should remain dry; you should not handle it with wet hands or wet utensils. To draw out the fragrance before adding to the POTpourri jar, pound the whole spices with a mortar and pestle very lightly (not enough to break them up), then add immediately to the glass jar.

3. Add cured cannabis flowers to the middle ⅓ of the jar, on top of the spices, and leave the top ⅓ as air space. Close the jar tightly and gently shake until the herbs and spices are evenly distributed around the cannabis flowers.

Sometimes it is necessary to add a humidity-control packet to the POTpourri jar if an environment is more humid. This will not usually be an issue if you open the POTpourri jar once every few days, give it a shake, and allow it to breathe for an hour or so. The longer you store your POTpourri, the more the cannabis flowers will infuse with fragrance and flavor.

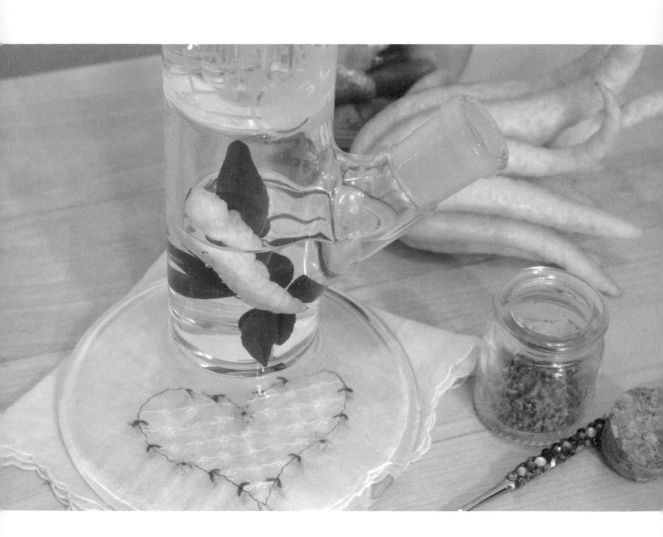

Flower and Fruit Essence Technique for Your Bubbler

any combination of fresh flowers, herbs, or fruit*

a glass bowl filled with spring or purified water

a sunny day outside or a warm sunny indoor windowsill**

a small mesh filter or screen***

Essence waters are a "living" water made with fresh flowers, herbs, and fruits, as opposed to distilled floral hydrosols such as rose water or orange flower water.

The technique for creating a whole living water essence has been in use for hundreds of years and is quite simple. An example of the living water essence technique is the Bach Flower Remedy. The technique in this book differs from the Bach method in that it's not a homeopathic dilution and instead contains the full aroma and taste of the flowers, herbs, and fruits that are used to make the water.

1. Place all of the plant material in the bowl and press down the plant material a few times to gently bruise the material so it begins to release essential flavors and fragrances. Pour water over the plant material until completely covered. You may add stone weights if necessary to keep the plant material submerged. Put this in a very warm and sunny place for 3 hours or more.

2. Strain the plant material from the essence water and store essence water in the refrigerator for up to 48 hours. It's best to add a dash of citric acid or lemon juice to maintain its freshness. It's ready to use in your bubbler as soon as it is strained from the plant material, but it's even more delicious when chilled first!

---

* My favorite combination is sliced oranges and fresh roses.

** I prefer a windowsill indoors that gets a few hours of direct sun.

*** The strainer shouldn't block sunlight, but should keep out debris and insects if you are putting the bowl outside to extract.

Bubbler Aromatherapy with Floral and Herbal Hydrosol
Commercially available floral and herbal water, or hydrosol, is another way to enjoy an aromatherapeutic experience with your bubbler. Hydrosols are commonly available in ethnic grocers or natural-food stores. Some of the more common varieties are rose water, orange flower water, and mint water. Choose one that does not contain preservatives and keep it refrigerated when not in use.
   Add 1 part hydrosol to 5 parts plain water for a more intense flavor and aroma.
   Drop this down to 10 parts plain water (or greater dilution) for more subtle effects.
If your bubbler has ice pinches, use them! Ice and chilled water enhance the experience even more!

Stay Hydrated with Spa Water!

Cannabis is a drawing and drying herb. For this reason, your indulgent cannabis spa day should include the best hydration method—chilled spa water. Prepare these in a large glass dispenser and include ice. I've made these in a gallon size and refrigerated them for up to 3 days.

Rooh Afza Spa Water

This is my signature spa water for cannabis spa day! It is based on a Pakistani beverage of the same name which is a proprietary herbal squash formula to treat the effects of very hot and dry environmental conditions on the human body. Rooh Afza syrup, used to make beverages and even ice cream, is widely available at Indian and Middle Eastern shops under various brand names.

My recipe includes many of the same cooling fruits, flowers, and herbs included in the original formula in a new recipe that is just for spa water.

cut citrus blends*
floral blend of roses and/
    or citrus blossoms**
green herb blend of mint,
    citrus leaves, lemon
    balm, or lemongrass
melon blend of
    watermelon,
    honeydew, or
    cantaloupe

1. In a gallon-sized glass container, fill ¼ of the way with your favorite combination of these cooling fruits, flowers, and herbs, paying special attention to creating a top note with rose, which is the centerpiece of this cooling spa water.
2. Fill the container over halfway with ice cubes or chips, leaving about ⅓ at the top for filling with water.
3. As the ice melts, the essential oils and flavors will be released from the ingredients—leave this out and enjoy it all day long!

---

* Use blood orange, citron, and lemon, but avoid grapefruit or bitter citrus.

** Orange and lemon blossoms work well.

Southern Peach Spa Water

cut oranges and lemons
cut peaches
mint leaves

This spa water was inspired by the sweltering heat and the divine peaches of the southern states! This cooling spa water recipe is designed to cut through the heat and is great for workouts and yoga, too.

1. In a gallon-sized glass container fill ¼ of the way with cut oranges, lemons, peaches, and mint, paying special attention to creating a top note with peach, which is the centerpiece of this cooling spa water. Use very firm peaches for best results with this spa water recipe.
2. Fill the container over halfway with ice cubes or chips, leaving about ⅓ at the top for filling with water.
3. As the ice melts, the essential oils and flavors will be released from the ingredients—leave this out and enjoy it all day long!

Tea, Bhang, and Smoothies

Try some delicious nosh for your spa day that's rich in nutritious hemp protein!

Apothecary Cannabis Rose Chai*

A sublime chai that you will fall in love with; this is a rose garden in a tea cup.

I've always dreamed of growing cannabis in a rose garden, and this lovely chai is as close as I've come to capturing that dream in a single recipe. I hope you'll love it as much as I do!

Makes four servings

1. Prepare two pans on the stove, one to contain the tea ingredients, and the other to contain the cannabis milk.
2. In the first pan for the tea, put 1 cup (240 milliliters) water in the pan along with the rose petals, black tea, broken cardamom pod, and cinnamon stick. Heat the water until it boils, then remove from heat and allow to steep while preparing the cannabis milk.
3. In the second pan, simmer the cannabis and coconut milk together on medium low for 15 minutes.
4. Remove the cannabis coconut milk from the stove and strain evenly into individual cups.
5. Add the rose water to the pan with the warm tea ingredients, then strain into individual cups. Follow by straining the cannabis milk evenly into each cup with the cannabis coconut milk. Serve immediately.

2 cups (480 milliliters) coconut milk
1 tablespoon (1 gram) rose petals
1 tablespoon (2 grams) black tea
1 green cardamom pod
1 cinnamon stick
1 gram or more potent cannabis flowers, finely ground
1 tablespoon (15 grams) demerara
OR other natural sugar or sugar-free sweetener to taste
¼ cup (60 milliliters) rose water

---

* Contains THC

Soothing Tummy Tea Bhang*

2 cups (480 milliliters) water

½ cup (100 grams) thinly sliced or shredded fresh ginger root

1 gram or more potent cannabis flowers, finely ground

1 tablespoon (15 milliliters) coconut oil or grass-fed ghee

½ cup (120 grams) shelled raw hemp seed

1 tablespoon (15 grams) demerara *OR* natural sugar or sugar-free sweetener to taste

This bhang recipe is so simple, yet so effective for upset tummies! Ginger is featured prominently in this recipe. I recommend that you get it fresh and slice/shred it yourself for the best results.

Makes four servings

1. Prepare two pans on the stove, one to contain the ginger tea, and the other to contain the cannabis milk.

2. In the first pan for the tea, put 1 cup (240 milliliters) of water in the pan along with the sliced or shredded ginger. Heat until it boils and remove from heat and allow to steep while preparing the cannabis milk.

3. In the second pan, heat the cannabis and oil or ghee on low for 10 minutes. Alternatively, if you already have some pre-prepared cannabis coconut oil or ghee—"cannabutter"— you may skip this step and melt enough to serve four people, and add it directly to the warm hemp milk.

4. In the blender, add 1 cup (240 milliliters) of water, hemp seed, and sugar, and blend until milky. Add this to the cannabis and oil in the pan and stir frequently, holding the temperature around 300 degrees Fahrenheit (150 degree Celsius) for 5 minutes. Remove from heat.

5. Strain the ginger tea into each cup, strain the cannabis milk evenly into each cup, then top with enough hot water to fill each cup and serve.

---

* Contains THC

European Cannabis Sipping Chocolate*

A thick, dark chocolate drink perfect for holiday entertaining or any time! Float fresh raspberries on the finished chocolate or dust with cinnamon for the finishing touch.

Makes four servings

1. In a pan on the stove, heat the cannabis and the oil or ghee on low heat for 10 minutes. Alternatively, if you already have some pre-prepared cannabis coconut oil or ghee—"cannabutter"—you may skip this step and melt enough to serve four people, and add it directly to the warm hemp milk.
2. In a blender, combine the water, hemp seed, cacao, vanilla, and sugar until smooth.
3. Return the pan with the cannabis and oil or ghee mixture to the stove and pour in the hemp chocolate mixture. Heat to 300 degrees Fahrenheit (150 degrees Celsius) for about 5 minutes.
4. Serve immediately in small, European-style chocolate cups.

1 gram or more potent cannabis flowers, finely ground
1 tablespoon (15 milliliters) coconut oil or grass-fed ghee
2 cups (480 milliliters) water
1 cup (250 grams) shelled raw hemp seed
3 tablespoons (15 grams) raw powdered cacao
1 teaspoon (5 milliliters) vanilla extract
3 tablespoons (45 grams) demerara *OR* natural sugar or sugar-free sweetener to taste

---

* Contains THC

Mango Hemp Lassi*

2 large (4 small) mangoes,
 peeled and sliced
1 cup (250 grams) shelled
 raw hemp seed
1 teaspoon (5 milliliters)
 vanilla extract
1 cup (240 milliliters)
 seltzer water, chilled
1 cup (250 grams) ice
 chips or cubes
1 dash black salt**
1 dash cinnamon

—————
* Does NOT contain THC

—————
** This is optional, but very
good and the secret to a great
mango lassi!

It is thought that mango potentiates the effects of cannabis, which makes this the perfect smoothie to enjoy while soaking in a cannabis bath or after a massage with a topical lotion or balm. This mango lassi is vegan and has 10 grams of protein per serving.

Makes four servings

Everything goes straight into the blender. Blend until creamy and smooth. Serve immediately.

Hemp New York Egg Cream*

3 tablespoons (15 grams)
 raw cacao powder
1 tablespoon (15 milliliters)
 vanilla extract
1½ cups (370 grams)
 shelled raw hemp seed
¼ cup (60 grams)
 demerara
 OR natural sugar or
 sugar-free sweetener
 to taste
2 cups (480 milliliters)
 chilled seltzer or
 sparkling water, chilled
1 cup (250 grams) ice
 chips or cubes

—————
* Does NOT contain THC

A classic fountain favorite—the New York Egg Cream—is loved by grownups and kids everywhere! This version has a wealth of protein and nutrients, which makes it a really smart sweet treat or snack any time.

Makes four servings

Put everything into the blender, and blend until it becomes a frothy milk with a "head." Pour into glasses and serve with a straw!

Blood Orange Hemp Cream Smoothie*

Another wintry favorite perfect for the holidays or Valentine's Day. Its pretty pink color comes from the blood orange, which has a berry-orange flavor totally unique to this variety of orange. It's packed with 10 grams of protein per serving, too!

Makes four servings

Everything goes straight into the blender. Blend until creamy and smooth. Serve immediately.

1 quart (1 liter) freshly squeezed blood orange juice
2 large bananas
2 teaspoons (10 milliliters) vanilla extract
1 cup (250 grams) ice chips or cubes
1 cup (250 grams) shelled raw hemp seed

---

* Does NOT contain THC

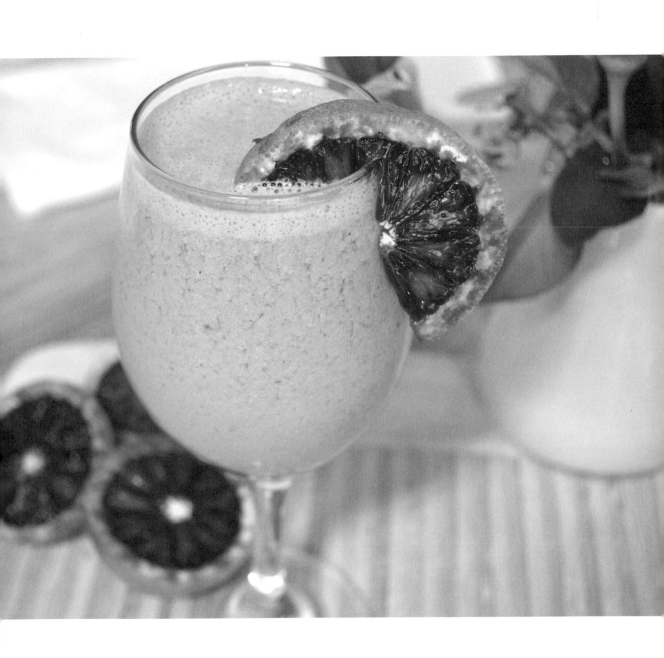

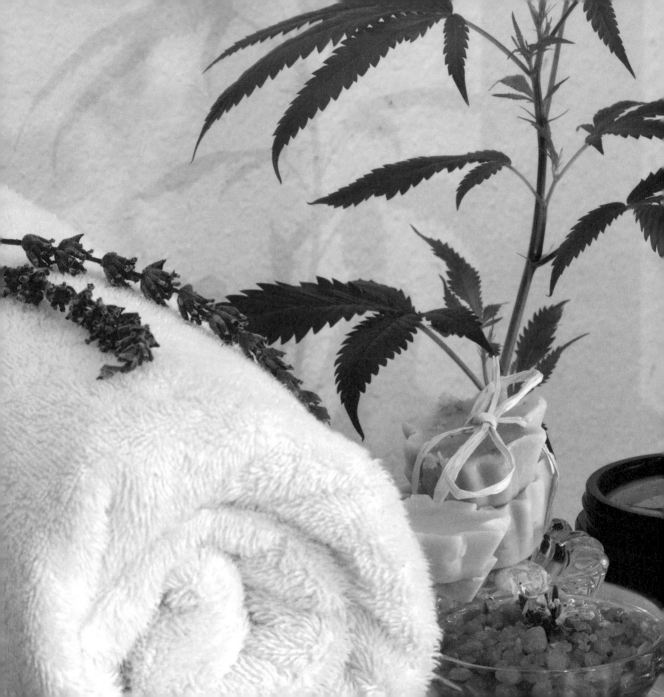

CONCLUSION AND RESOURCE GUIDE

In this section, I've included my favorite ingredient and tool resources for making every recipe in this book. Nothing in this section is a paid endorsement—these are brands and shops that I personally patronize, as I'm very satisfied with the quality of the ingredients they carry.

Natural Foods Stores and Amazon.com
Hands down the best two places to find almost every ingredient or tool you will need to to make the recipes in this book.

Natur-Oli Soapberries | naturoli.com
My favorite brand of soapberry and the one I chose for making the cannabis bath bases. Their soapberries are very fresh and organic. Natur-Oli sells their soapberries on Amazon, but they often have great deals in their own online shop, so check that out, too.

Eden Botanicals | edenbotanicals.com
One of the best sources out there for solvent-free aromatherapy-grade essential oils. They also offer many of the rarer and more expensive essential oils for sale in sample-drop sizes that are very budget-friendly if you'd like to try your hand experimenting with high-quality essential oils.

Camden Grey | camdengrey.com
This is a reliable source for many of the high in oleic acid plant butters I use to formulate my spa creations. They also have great customer service and include free samples with every order.

Lekithos Inc. | mysunflowerlecithin.com
Sunflower lecithin is used generously throughout the recipes in this book for its superior emulsifying properties and health benefits. Lekithos is a truly solvent-free and GMO-free sunflower lecithin that I use and recommend.

Your Local Ethnic Supermarket
Many of the recipes in this book use ingredients that are quite common in ethnic Indian and Middle Eastern supermarkets, including oils, spices, and fresh herbs.

Mehandi Henna | Mehandi.com
The only online store where I've been able to find real henna flower essential oil. A $10 vial will make many recipes in this book!

RECIPE INDEX

INDEX